The Neuroscience of Everyday Life

Sam Wang, Ph.D.

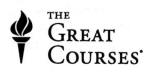

THE
GREAT
COURSES®

PUBLISHED BY:

THE GREAT COURSES
Corporate Headquarters
4840 Westfields Boulevard, Suite 500
Chantilly, Virginia 20151-2299
Phone: 1-800-832-2412
Fax: 703-378-3819
www.thegreatcourses.com

Sam Wang, Ph.D.

Associate Professor of Molecular Biology
and Neuroscience, Princeton University

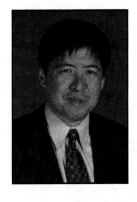

Professor Sam Wang is Associate Professor of Molecular Biology and Neuroscience at Princeton University. He was born to immigrant parents in Cincinnati, Ohio, and moved to Riverside, California, with them, one brother, and one sister. In 1986, at the age of 19, he received his B.S. in Physics with honor at the California Institute of Technology, making him the youngest member of his graduating class. In 1994, he earned his Ph.D. in Neurosciences at Stanford University School of Medicine, where he did his research at the Hopkins Marine Station in Pacific Grove, California. His research concerned the signaling properties of calcium, a universal signaling ion in all cells, including neurons. His current research uses advanced optical methods to probe brain circuit function, with a focus on the cerebellum's role in perception, movement, and higher cognitive function.

After his doctoral research, Professor Wang continued his research at Duke University Medical Center, where he turned his attention to the molecular mechanisms by which neurons signal to one another using neurotransmitters. At this time he was a Grass Fellow in Neurophysiology at the Marine Biological Laboratory in Woods Hole, Massachusetts. It was also during this time that he was selected by the American Association for the Advancement of Science (AAAS) as a Congressional Science and Engineering Fellow. He spent a year away from the lab, on the staff of the U.S. Senate Committee on Labor and Human Resources. He handled reauthorization of the National Science Foundation and tracked federal education, science, and technology policy and budget trends for the late Senator Edward M. Kennedy. He also coordinated Mass NetDay96, a government-education-private partnership to bring Internet infrastructure to hundreds of public schools in Massachusetts.

After his work at Duke and on Capitol Hill, in 1997 Professor Wang moved to Bell Labs Lucent Technologies, where he worked as a postdoctoral member of the technical staff in the Physics Research Laboratory. With David Tank and Winfried Denk, he worked on the development and use of new technologies for probing living neural tissue by using multiphoton optical methods. After a brief stint at the Max Planck Institute for Medical Research in Heidelberg, Germany, he joined the faculty of Princeton University as an Assistant Professor in 2000 and was promoted to Associate Professor in 2006.

Professor Wang's research has resulted in the publication of more than 50 papers in leading peer-reviewed journals, including *Nature*, *Nature Neuroscience*, *Proceedings of the National Academy of Sciences*, *Neuron*, *Journal of Neuroscience*, and *Public Library of Science ONE*. He has won numerous awards for his research, including an Alfred P. Sloan Fellowship, the Rita Allen Foundation Young Scholars Fellowship, a Distinguished Young Investigator Award from the W. M. Keck Foundation, and a CAREER Award from the National Science Foundation. His research findings span from the function of single synapses to the architecture of whole brains. His work includes the discovery that learning mechanisms can, in the first minutes of the process, act like all-or-none switches, and that bird and mammalian brains share similar architectures for generating complex social relations. He is also known for innovative use of optical methods for probing the neural function of living brain tissue, both in vitro and in awake, behaving animals, by using multiphoton microscopy and light-sensitive "caged" neurotransmitters. His research has been featured on National Public Radio and in *The New York Times*.

In addition to his scientific research, Professor Wang is known for his public communication in the areas of neuroscience and statistics. In 2004 he pioneered the use of statistical meta-analysis to model the U.S. presidential election, establishing a method of polling analysis that was elaborated by dozens of hobbyists worldwide in 2004 and 2008. In 2008 he founded the Princeton Election Consortium, which came within 1 electoral vote of estimating the final outcome of the presidential race. This web-based modeling project attracted more than a million viewers and was featured on Fox News and in *The Wall Street Journal*.

Professor Wang is co-author with Sandra Aamodt of a bestselling popular book on neuroscience, *Welcome to Your Brain: Why You Lose Your Car Keys but Never Forget How to Drive and Other Puzzles of Everyday Life*. The book has been translated into more than 20 languages worldwide and was recipient of the AAAS/Subaru Science Book of the Year Award in the Young Adult category. He has written extensively for general audiences in *The New York Times*, *The Washington Post*, *USA Today*, and the *New York Daily News*. He speaks often to public audiences and to the media on neuroscience and on his research. He has been profiled in *The New York Times* and made appearances on National Public Radio and the TED^{x}SF and Big Think online video series.

Professor Wang lives in Princeton, New Jersey, with his wife, who is a physician; their daughter; and a pug. ∎

Table of Contents

Table of Contents

The Neuroscience of Everyday Life

Scope:

For millennia, people have been interested in the workings of their own minds. This interest has found expression in disciplines as diverse as philosophy, medicine, and psychology. Today, neuroscience addresses the mind as arising from the brain, a biological organ. Brains mediate our daily experiences at every level, from breathing and sleeping to making decisions, loving, and learning. Neuroscience is starting to provide explanations for every aspect of behavior. Tens of thousands of neuroscientists now examine brain function at levels ranging from molecules to cells to circuits to the whole brain. Although neuroscience is often taught in terms of disease, this is an excessively limited view. We use our brains in our every action. Understanding the brain can illuminate our daily lives—and what it means to be an individual person.

The brain is an ever-changing biological organ

Popular belief has it that the brain is like a computer. The brain processes information, but beyond that, the analogy does not hold up well. Everyday experiences reveal ways in which your brain operates in a most un-computerlike fashion. Examples include visual illusions, the emotional basis of decision-making, irrational approaches to problem-solving, and the unreliability of human memory. These phenomena reflect the evolutionary history of the brain, which has been optimized by natural selection to help you live to fight another day and to reproduce. Even unusual capacities, such as humor and mathematics, are reflected by similar capacities in other animals.

A brain's entire activity consumes only about as much energy as an idling laptop. Brain cells make trillions of connections with one another. Some connections come from the external world, bringing in coded signals that drastically condense the available information. These signals are reconstituted by mechanisms in the brain—but never with absolute certainty.

The brain changes throughout life. Many changes are preprogrammed in early development, which proceeds normally except in cases of flawed genetic inheritance or severe deprivation. The interplay of genes, environment, and experience continues throughout life. From childhood to old age, active use of skills plays a major role in maintaining and enhancing function. As a biological organ, the brain is vulnerable to cardiovascular disease—and is kept healthy by physical exercise, which helps the brain retain function and can alleviate the symptoms of anxiety and depression.

A second type of change in the brain depends on experience: memory. The brain's many forms of memory each use different brain regions. The capacity to remember facts relies on the medial temporal lobe system for memory, which also handles spatial navigation; many memory tricks rely on this commonality. Memory is fluid: Information that seems to be permanently stored undergoes constant change as memories are reprocessed and consolidated, so that a decades-old memory may be vivid yet lack detail or context.

Unusual and altered states

Our brain reacts to many extreme experiences with the stress response, which temporarily conserves resources. But persistent stress can have unhealthy effects on the growth and birth of neurons. Modern life includes work, a source of chronic stress, but also play, which triggers short-term responses, such as the secretion of adrenalin, but without creating a long-term stress burden.

The brain typically represents the body in a seamless fashion, but exceptional events can occur. Pain can even be felt in an extremity after it has been amputated, a syndrome that is caused by lingering representations in the brain. Under extreme conditions, people often report incredible events, such as out-of-body and near-death experiences. Paranormal events may be caused by seizures or insult to the temporal-parietal junction, a site where body image is represented.

Humans have found ways to alter the brain's function chemically. Mind-altering drugs are as diverse as nicotine, Prozac, morphine, and caffeine. Both legal and illegal drugs work by enhancing or interfering with the function of protein molecules that process neurotransmitter signals. Receptors for a particular neurotransmitter can often be found all over the brain, leading to side effects—sometimes catastrophic ones—such as addiction.

The individual, social, and spiritual brain

Brain variations establish our individual characteristics. Some differences are small, such as those between men and women, who differ most in sexual behavior not cognitive ability. Human variation in personality and cognitive capacity is built on genetic foundations; therefore, we share many such traits with our parents. Differences in cognitive ability are also seen across generations, a period during which the environment's influence on development changes tremendously.

Humans are intensely social animals and are able to imagine the mental states of others. This capacity provides a key component for many group dynamics, including religious belief. One component of this "theory of mind" capacity may reside in the insula, which is active in processing both one's own emotional state and that of others—and perhaps provides a means for feeling sympathy for others. Insight into theory of mind may come from autism, a genetically based developmental disorder in which social reasoning is impaired.

Some areas of mental function are only beginning to be probed. One example is the basis of life happiness. Because of our ability to adapt to changing circumstances, major life events, including blindness and losing a limb, do not affect long-term happiness. Yet other life events have a lasting effect on happiness, such as gaining a life partner—or losing one. An exciting frontier is the understanding of both happiness and mood, which are profoundly affected by regions in the brain's core. These questions present a major challenge for neuroscience and its relation to everyday life. ■

The Mozart Myth and Active Learning
Lecture 19

Think of it as like this: When you're building a house, you can decide where you want to arrange the bedrooms. You can decide exactly where you want the windows and so on. But once the house has been built, changes are harder. You can rearrange the furniture or replace the furniture, but the floor plan is set.

Many parents fret over whether their young children can learn to excel without a roster of extracurricular activities, but it's important to realize that many aspects of brain development are preprogrammed and don't require anything beyond normal experiences. Further, most environments are sufficient for normal development. The key principles of early mental development don't include extraordinary learning activities, just active engagement and age-appropriate experiences.

In utero, the brain requires no experiences at all, because it's busy growing large numbers of nonselective neurons, forming axons, and migrating neurons to final destinations. After this process of explosive growth, the brain begins to edit itself. In the first two years of life, neurons that aren't used die and are removed, a regressive process.

There is some evidence that, during those important first years, intellectual ability may be enhanced by exposure to intellectually stimulating activities. For example, the IQ scores of children up to age 3 correlate with the number of words they hear each day, with higher scores related to the greater number of words heard. When these children are tested again in third grade, the correlation remains. In another example of active engagement, children who learn to play a musical instrument have better spatial reasoning skills than those who don't take music lessons. The engagement and practice of a skill is more likely to trigger active neuronal firing, leading to better development. Parents should encourage children to be active producers, not passive consumers.

The Flynn effect describes the steady increase in IQ scores in children in industrialized countries since World War II, pointing to the idea that better nutrition and a more complex, stimulating environment (including more social interaction, thanks to improved mass communication) may enhance brain development. This trend has leveled off in recent years.

Active engagement is effective in teaching certain skills or concepts only when the brain is ready to learn that specific skill or concept. Some forms of brain plasticity are no longer available after a certain age. For example, a scientist blinded in childhood but restored to

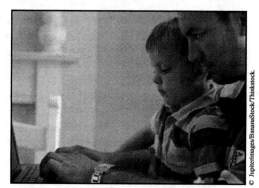

Children today have a more intellectually stimulating environment than those of 100 years ago.

sight through surgery in adulthood had trouble distinguishing shadows from objects; he finally got a seeing-eye dog. He missed some critical context early in life, when the brain was ready to learn what a shadow was versus an object.

Another age-appropriate experience is acquiring language, best done before age 6. Early learners of multiple languages learn to speak as natives with no accent. The Broca's area of the brain (the brain region that produces speech) in multilingual children lights up no matter which language is spoken; for adult learners, other areas light up for the later-acquired language. The window for learning accent closes sooner than for learning grammar, both for spoken languages and for signed languages: Hand movements that are not entirely natural seem to correspond to the sign language equivalent of having an accent. ■

1. What are the roles of passive and active experience in shaping brain development?

2. What does the per-generation rate of the Flynn effect tell you about the role of genes and environment in brain development? How might this limit what we can say about the innate abilities of a particular group, such as a race?

The Mozart Myth and Active Learning
Lecture 19—Transcript

Welcome back. In the last lecture we considered the way in which infants are ready to learn from a very early age and how they interpret their new experiences as they come into the world. Let's follow those infants into childhood and think about what they are experiencing as they a little bit older.

Here are the themes that I'd like to talk about today about how children can be influenced by their experiences and how changes in babies and children are preprogrammed. So in fact, what I I'm going to do is go back in development a little bit and talk about the programs that establish the development of the brain, and how these programs only require normal experience, not enhanced experience such as enhanced preschool programs, that sort of thing.

That having been said, I'll also talk about the environmental programs that can influence cognitive development in children. I'll talk about windows of opportunity, windows of time during children's development for some experiences to arrive, during which those experiences need to arrive in order for development to proceed normally. Along the way, I'll give you replacements for this Mozart Myth that we've been talking about.

Recall that I described the Mozart Myth, we'll come back to it one more time, the idea that playing classical music to babies increases their intelligence. This belief has made major inroads into popular awareness and one way of thinking about is, it's a way that people think that they can get something for nothing. You can park your kid in front of some music or a baby DVD and he'll get smarter.

To be fair, the Baby Mozart, Baby Einstein Myth plays into a natural desire to improve our children, and so it is a desire that we have to do things to help our children. Before you get too carried away with that kind of thinking, you should know that, in fact, there is a wide range of normal experience, I'll give you an example, a wide range of experience that can lead to adequate outcomes.

As a child, I spent hours each day watching television. I watched terrible, terrible television. I watched all kinds of stuff. There are certain things I just watched over and over again. For instance, I can still recite the plot of almost every episode of the original Star Trek series or The Brady Bunch. This is the way I spent a lot of my childhood. It turns out that I seemed to have found gainful employment that involves using my brain, so apparently, there was not too much damage involved with that. So, that is an example of some of the enrichment that I got when I was a kid.

This leads in to a major point that I want to make about the kind of input and the kind of environment that's necessary for infant and early childhood development. It turns out that a lot of infant and early childhood development proceeds on its own. Most environments, as long as they're normal, are sufficient for development and are sufficient for normal development. It is true that deprivation can interfere with brain development. So for example, there is a well-known example of children who spent the early years in orphanages in Romania. It turns out that orphanages in Romania had a policy of just having kids in a crib, left alone for years, visited only by a caretaker who came along once in awhile to change diapers. Those children ended up having lifelong problems and had difficulties with language, acquiring social skills, and living a normal life. That's an example of deprivation in early life being necessary for abnormal development.

Unless you're locking your kid in a closet, which I definitely encourage you to stop doing, unless you're doing that, there is no risk of this kind of outcome. So, that's an example of normal experience being sufficient over a wide range of possibilities in leading children to develop relatively normally.

So, let's go back to normal development. In the last lecture we learned that as early as three months of age, babies have demonstrated mechanisms for learning from their environments. Before that, though, before the age of three months, earlier stages of their development did not require experience at all. And that's a good thing because many of those stages happen while the mother is pregnant before birth, where there is not really that much stimulation available. So these early stages operate according to programs that more or less operate on their own. These events include events such as the following. During neural development, during brain development, the different areas of the brain form, neurons are born and then they migrate to their final positions, as neurons take their positions in the nervous system. Then axons grow out to their intended targets, sometimes over long distances, so that neurons can send axons out to them and some innervation to project into other parts of the brain.

These parts of the process can go wrong. It is possible for drugs or toxins in the mother's body or genetic mutations in the fetus to drive the process in a wrong direction. In those cases, severe birth defects often can result. Under normal circumstances this process proceeds by itself, on its own. This stage of brain development is sufficient to permit many basic behaviors, such as withdrawal from a rapidly approaching object. So there are a few simple things that the developing brain can do.

What does early experience do to the brain? We talked about this a little bit before in the context of what babies are ready to learn. After the baby is born, sensory experience starts to become important. We talked about it a little bit before. Sensory experience starts to become important for some aspects of brain development. In any normal environment, most of the necessary experience is easily available. So we don't, for instance, need to send our kids to vision enrichment camp. Kids learn how to see simply from looking at the world around them.

Given what I've told you, you might imagine that sensory experience is like fertilizer for growing connections. It's sort of like watering a plant. Maybe you just need to give a little sensory experience and, perhaps, maybe sensory experience directs axons to grow into specific places. Maybe there is some sensory experience that says, "Okay, it's time for you to make a connection."

However, it turns out to be the reverse. It turns out to be not like that at all. There is a general brain principle. The general brain principle is that early development involves two kinds of steps, one kind of step which is a growth process, another kind of step which involves regressive processes. So roughly speaking, one can think of early developmental events as being progressive, so for instance, neurons being born or axons forming the way I

9

described. You can also think of regressive events. So neurons can die and axons can be removed. This is a second type of process that you would not imagine as being a central part of development. It turns out that, in fact, the brain produces a huge number of relatively nonselective connections between neurons, say between one area and another area. Then there is this large number of nonselective connections arising during early development. Then what happens is that the ones that aren't being used are removed over the first two years of life, at least in our species. We can think of the necessary role of sensory experience as perhaps playing more of a role like pruning, as opposed to triggering growth.

I've told you that experience expectant development is part of normal development. It's also important for the development of a child's intelligence. I've given you the extreme example of deprivation of the Romanian orphanages. There is some evidence that intellectual ability may be enhanced by exposure to intellectually stimulating activities, what we often call "enrichment." This is something that, of course, has some practical applications. It's worth looking at the evidence to think carefully about just how much influence we have over our children's intellectual development, and how much of it is things that we can do purposefully such as sending a kid to music camp or what have you, or something that just comes from the environment in ways that are perhaps harder for us to control.

Let's think of a few examples. Here is the first thing that one might do as a scientist. One might look in animals, laboratory animals, and ask, if you enriched the environment of a laboratory animal, does it help the mental function of those animals? Here is an experiment that has been done. Mice that are housed with other mice, to give them a social environment, and an assortment of toys that are changed frequently, have larger brains, have larger neurons, have more glial cells, the support cells that surround neurons, and more synapses than mice that are just housed alone in standard cages. So these are things that can be seen experimentally. These enriched animals, let's call them "enriched," also learned to complete a variety of tasks more easily. These tasks are improved not only in young mice, but also in adult and old mice as well. So this enrichment effect occurs at different ages.

You might imagine, okay, well enrichment is apparently good for the brains of lab mice, but can it be applied to humans? There is an ambiguity. The ambiguity is, what does it mean to enrich a lab animal compared with enriching the life of, say, a human child? How enriched are we compared with lab animals? Lab animals live in a very simplified environment. A typical lab animal has a pretty boring life. The cage is not complicated, so there is no navigation through complicated places to look for food or look for other animals who might be suitable mates. There is no applying to college. There are no college application essays to write. It's really pretty simple there in the cage. One objection to the result being interpreted as being supportive of the role of enrichment is that this research might not be so much about the positive effects of enrichment on the brain, but about the negative effects of deprivation in the typical laboratory environment. What they suggest is the possibility that we don't yet know exactly what the normal range of experience is for lab animals. There is some difficulty with interpreting this evidence from lab animals.

There is another set of evidence that comes from studying human children growing up in their home environments. This piece of evidence is a little bit more interesting because it starts to speak to our experience. Investigators have looked at a number of factors in the first three years of life, parenting features, such as how parents talk to their children and the number of words that a child hears. One very interesting observation that has come out of this work is that the number of words that a small child hears per day, before the age of three, is correlated with IQ. It's correlated with IQ measured at the age of three, but of course, one argument as well, you're not really measuring IQ, whatever IQ is. What you're measuring is what that kid has learned in that first 36 months.

It turns out that these measures of parenting, such as number of words heard per day, are also correlated with IQ in third grade, so it's something that's measurable six or seven years later. That's very interesting because that's an observation that holds up, even after controlling for other factors such as race and socioeconomic status. What it suggests is the possibility that there is something about environmental influences, such as the number of words heard per day and the complexity of a child's verbal environment, that could, in fact, affect a child's cognitive development. So there is some possibility that environment may have some influence on children's development.

There is another line of evidence that's interesting that suggests an environmental role. In this case, it's an environmental role that's not necessarily within the control of parents. It's a very interesting effect that was discovered some years ago called "the Flynn Effect." And the Flynn Effect was, of course, named after a person named Flynn. The person named Flynn in this case is James R. Flynn, who is a philosopher and political scientist, and he also turns out to be an excellent statistical analyst.

What Flynn did was gather data obtained by other investigators in their studies. What he did was he studied data from 20 countries from around the world. He did was he examined performance on standardized IQ tests over time. What he found was very interesting. These results go back actually 100 years, but the results are most strong in the period following World War II. So, let's talk about that.

What Professor Flynn found was that average IQ scores were steadily higher and higher for people who were born in later years. What he specifically found in industrialized countries, in developed countries, is that IQ scores increased by about three points per decade. He found some fairly extreme examples in some countries. The most extreme cases were Denmark and Israel. In these countries, IQ scores rose even faster, about 20 points over 30 years. That's little more than a single generation when you think about it, 20 points over 30 years. For example, in verbal and performance IQ, an average Danish 12-year-old in 1982 beat the average scores of a 14-year-old from his parent's generation in 1952. So that's children who were two years older from his parent's generation.

We look at these changes and it leads to one kind of question that sometimes comes up, which is, is the brain evolving? This is something that I often get asked. Could it possibly be that our brains are evolving over time? Well, clearly our species is subject to natural selection, and it's possible over long periods of time for a selection to occur. But in this particular case, in the case of the Flynn Effect, the answer is basically no. The reason goes like this. This is not enough time. This is within one generation, steady change over just a few decades. That's not enough time for evolution through natural selection, which requires genes to be passed on to offspring and then leading to one more round of reproduction and selection. So the fact that these things happened on a timescale of just a few decades is far too short for natural selection to occur.

So, what does that leave? What it leaves is environment. Evidently intelligence tests, which we think of as measuring some pure, inborn capacity, IQ, it turns out that these intelligence tests evidently don't just measure some pure, inborn capacity. They seem to also track the effects of the environmental surroundings in which a person matures. That's interesting. The environment can affect measured IQ.

How could this be? Well, it's possible to think of a few reasons. One possibility is that better nutrition and health can lead to better brain growth. It could be that, for instance, in the period following World War II, food which was short before, was not in abundance, became more abundant in many countries and that led to better brain growth in children.

Another possibility is that the environment has gotten more complex. This is one that Professor Flynn subscribes to, the idea that over in his argument, the last 100 years a more stimulating environment may enhance brain development and function, and may reward the kinds of functions that are important in modern society, such as abstract reasoning. The argument goes like this. If we compare a preindustrial society and even a society during the industrial revolution with what children in developed countries now grow up with, children now have a much more intellectually stimulating environment and much better nutrition. We think about all the factors that are available now in developed countries: standardized schooling, better nutrition, mass entertainment—for what it's worth, with all the information that comes in from mass entertainment—computers, cell phones, other technology. These are all things that were not available just a few decades ago uniformly throughout society.

Furthermore, in addition to all these factors, it's possible to imagine that these factors may be intensified by social interaction with other individuals. Recall that I mentioned the observation that the number of words per day is associated with IQ years later. Well, one way to get words per day is social interaction with other individuals. If those other individuals are also developmentally accelerated, now we have a positive feedback effect so that when children are accelerated, other children are accelerated. They talk to one another and that's a positive feedback effect. That could lead to even more improved performance.

It's entirely possible that people's brains today are on average more sophisticated than they were 100 years ago. It's likely that that's not because of genetic reasons, not because of DNA-based reasons, but because of some changes in the environment. It seems to be the case that this effect may be starting to level off. For instance in Denmark, I mentioned Denmark as being one of the countries with the largest past gains, in recent years, IQ scores have stopped increasing. They have started to level off a bit.

Let's think about this a little bit more. Let's think about exactly how genes, how environment, could have an effect on brain development. One possibility that's the subject of an investigation that is supported by some evidence is that environmental effects can limit brain development. Think back to the Romanian orphanages. Imagine that we have a certain amount of potential when we're born and environment effects can limit our development when resources are scarce. So in other words, one way to explain the Flynn Effect is, as the number of people who are poor or resource deprived decreases in the world, then the average IQ increases. There is some support for this. There is a recent study of Spanish children who, like the Danish and Israeli and other children around the world, Spanish children showed intelligence gains in the population over a 30- year period. What was observed in these children is that IQ scores among the lowest scoring children went up the most, and there was hardly any gain in the top half of the population. So the bottom half of the population seemed to get better over that 30-year period, not the upper half.

If we think about this, it actually is also consistent with another observation that's made in the United States, and this observation has been made about what predicts achievement in schools. It has been observed that at poorer levels of society educational achievement is correlated with the resources available in schools. So if you're poor, then how much your schools have is important. But at a richer level of society, now educational achievement is more strongly correlated with heredity and home environment. So, in fact, this can even account for disagreements that occur politically when people say, well, it's home environment and it's my family. Well, it's the schools. In fact, both sides could in fact be right based on the evidence that's observed.

Now I've raised for you several different issues. Remember that I said in a previous lecture, briefly in the context of willpower, that IQ is hard to train. Now I've given you another observation, this Flynn Effect, and these effects of resources. So evidently, there is a degree to which IQ can be malleable by the environment. This even raises the possibility that I think by now has occurred to some of you, that environmental influences could have a large enough effect that we could see differences between groups, between socioeconomic groups, between racial groups.

And there's even evidence for this. And this is a very interesting piece of work. And Flynn has written about this. It's a work that was conducted by someone named Eiferth. This is a work in which the academic accomplishments of children were studied under a condition under which environmental factors were similar and taken out of racial context. The specific study was done on illegitimate babies fathered by occupying soldiers, so these are mostly American soldiers, some French soldiers, in Germany after World War II. These babies, some had white fathers and others had black fathers, but they were schooled together. What was observed is that these babies had nearly identical IQs despite their fathers coming from groups with different IQs back home. What seems to be the case is that this disappearance in racial differences points towards the possibility that race differences might, in fact, arise in part from environmental differences.

I'm going to turn to a different subject. Now I want to talk about the effects of experiences and when they're available. So far I've talked about experiences just being something that can affect the brain over development. In fact, that's not exactly right. Remember what I said in a previous lecture. I said that baby's brains are prepared to seek out certain experiences at defined developmental stages. I said that at three-months-of-age or at one-year-of-age, there are things that babies are ready to detect, such as correlations in syllables, that sort of thing, correlations in events. It turns out that there are certain times when such experiences can have a strong or permanent effect on the brain. There are windows of opportunity during which those experiences can have a very strong effect on the brain and not later. Those windows are called "sensitive periods."

So let's consider a few examples of sensitive periods. One example comes from a neuroscientist who, himself, experienced the effects of his missing a sensitive period during his own development. This is a neuroscientist named Mike May. He is a neuroscientist who was blinded as a child and he became a working scientist, but blind. As an adult, he had an operation that restored his sight. In principle, that's a wonderful thing to get back your sight. But it turned out that despite the fact that he had his sight back through this operation, he still had difficulties that were very hard to overcome. For example, he had difficult distinguishing shadows from objects. So, if he was walking along and he was walking down the street, he has difficulty distinguishing a shadow, from say, a rock, or a tree, or something like that.

It appears to be the case that he missed some critical context early in life, in which he learned what a shadow was versus an object. This has had consequences for him. So, for instance, despite being blind, he was an athlete and he is a competitive skier, a competitive blind skier. In fact, he had the downhill blind skiing record. So, when you ski downhill blind, you have to have someone guiding you, obviously. He held the record at 65 miles per hour with a guide. After regaining his sight through this operation, he one day was going down the slopes and encountered this large object, and he thought there was not time enough to stop. He thought for sure he was going to die. It turned out to be a shadow cast by a ski lift. This is an example of the kinds of difficulties that he experiences in daily life. He finds these difficulties to be quite distracting. For instance, now he does things like skis with his eyes closed, and he has a better time with that; because of now all the distractions that are constantly coming at him from the world, he now has acquired for the first time a seeing eye dog.

The lesson that we draw from this is that there is such a thing as age-appropriate experience. What has happened in the case of Mike May is that there was a period during his early development in which it would have been helpful to him to be able to learn about, say, shadows. He missed that experience.

Here is another example that perhaps has happened to many of you in your everyday lives. Now I want to cover the example of language acquisition. If you've ever tried to learn a language as an adult, or if you've met people who have learned a language as an adult, you may have noticed that these people are very likely to speak with an accent. It's possible to learn a language when you're older, but you perhaps will a language less thoroughly or in a different way. This is really characteristic of people who learn language as adults. The optimal time for acquiring language is far earlier than adulthood. It's before the age of six. In fact, children who learn languages before the age of six speak those languages as a native without any accent. So there is this period of time during which language, when acquired, is spoken naturally and idiomatically and is understood fluidly.

It turns out that when you look in the brains of these children, or if you look at the brains of people who speak multiple languages and learned them early in life, the representation of those languages in the brain overlap in the same brain area that is responsible for producing speech. This is the brain region in the frontal part of the brain known as "Broca's area." And the Broca's area represents languages. You can see the same part of the brain light up whether a person is speaking, say, English or French. That's not the case if people learn language later on. In that case, neighboring regions of the brain light up.

Interestingly, language acquisition doesn't seem to saturate in the sense that acquisition of individual languages is not slowed on average by the learning of multiple languages. For instance, if children learn multiple languages at once, they are still able to acquire languages as rapidly and without any particular problem. In fact, in some cases there are even ancillary benefits. So for example, in children who learn tonal languages such as Chinese, also in children who learn Japanese are Korean, children who learn those languages before the age of three are observed to have an increased likelihood of having absolute pitch, perfect pitch. So that's something that may be associated with the learning of language where children have to pay attention to tone.

Up to age seven or eight, children can still learn additional languages, and they can learn languages without noticeable problems. After the age of 12, children can learn language, but they never learn it fluently. This is true for spoken languages. It is even true for signed languages. It's possible to identify problems with grammar and accent in languages that are acquired after the age of 12. It's even possible to do this in the case of sign language. There is such a thing as hand movements that are not entirely natural that seem to correspond to the sign language equivalent of having an accent.

At some point, almost everyone reaches an age after which any new language is learned as a second language. In fact, I encountered this once when I met a colleague who is a Ph.D. scientist. He lived in the United States as a child and then moved to Germany. So he spoke English as a child in Germany. It was really quite odd talking with this guy because his pronunciation was perfect and idiomatic. He seemed like a natural English speaker, but his vocabulary was that of a child. It was really odd to encounter this in someone with a Ph.D. in my own field. It was an odd experience to talk with him because he sounded perfectly fine. In order to have a full-grown conversation with him, it was necessary to speak German, which I don't speak, unfortunately.

I'm going to sum up now what I've told you about sensitive periods; sensitive periods I will compare to an analogy of constructing a home. I've talked to you about periods of time when the brain is receptive to something. Think of it as like this. When you're building a house, you can decide where you want to arrange the bedrooms. You can decide exactly where you want the windows, and so on. But once the house has been built, changes are harder. You can rearrange the furniture or replace the furniture, but the floor plan is set.

In this analogy, let's go back to the language and the representation of languages, when children learn multiple languages, I mentioned that they are represented in the same region of the brain. That's not true for adults. I mentioned that in adults language is represented in adjacent areas. It's, as if to pursue the analogy a little bit further, as if to support language, we have to use the spare room.

There is a general principle here. The general principle here that comes from looking at Mike May, looking at language acquisition, is that different capabilities have different sensitive periods. What this means is that there is a time window in the case of language, for instance, for learning the sounds of language, and in the case of learning the language with an accent as opposed to without an accent, the time window for learning the sounds of a language tends to close earlier than the time window for learning grammar. What that suggests is that there are multiple forms of plasticity in the brain, multiple ways of learning, and we're back to learning again, that probably require different brain regions and probably change at different times over the course of development. In fact, this is related to laboratory observations. It's commonly observed in the laboratory that, for instance, synaptic plasticity, which we've talked about, or plasticity of neuronal structures such as the algorithm neurons and dendrites, that these forms of brain plasticity are greater at some ages and then the window closes. There are some forms of plasticity that are no longer possible after a certain age. So there is an analogous observation to the idea of sensitive periods behaviorally and in acquisition of skills over development at the level of synapses and circuits. So there seems to be something going on at multiple levels of activity. One major activity in neuroscience is to start linking these different kinds of sensitive periods.

I want to come back to the Mozart Effect. I've talked about the Mozart Effect a lot and I've been telling you about how the Mozart Effect is a source of problems and it's not true. I feel bad about that. I would like to now replace it with something a little bit better. It's unsurprising that there is no evidence for benefits for baby DVDs. Babies aren't ready for Mozart. The ability to use different kinds of information, of course, matures as I've told you, as brains become ready to process that information. It turns out that there is something that does work better than passive listening to Mozart and the thing that works better, of course later in childhood, and it's learning to play a musical instrument. Children who learn to play a musical instrument have better spatial reasoning skills than those who don't take music lessons. It may be because music and spatial reasoning are processed by similar brain systems, by overlapping brain regions. So a thing that you can do, rather than playing Mozart to a child passively, is to fill your house with music. Don't let the children be passive consumers. Make them be active producers.

Let's summarize what we've learned today. What we've learned is that many aspects of brain development are preprogrammed and only require normal experience. As I've mentioned in the previous and in this lecture, brains come ready to learn, but they come ready to learn at specific times. These sensitive periods are periods during which specific things find fertile ground in the brain. Plasticity mechanisms in the brain may also have sensitive time windows.

A common element of many of these observations is the difference between passive exposure and learning an active skill. Recall when I talked about memory mechanisms, I talked about Donald Hebb and the idea that cells that fire together wire together, and the engagement of an active skill, the practice of a skill, is more likely to trigger active neuronal firing. So there is something about active skill practice that leads to better development. So there are these key principles of early mental development. One is active engagement and the other is age appropriate experience.

In the next lecture what I'd like to do is continue development a little bit further; in the next lecture I want to start talking about adolescence.

Childhood and Adolescence
Lecture 20

Myelination is not complete until people reach their early 20s. Again, that suggests a possible physical basis for changes in self-control and changes in the ability to pay attention. So there is this sense that one gets from these changes in brain structure that there is a physical basis in the kinds of capacities that change as we go through adolescence and reach early adulthood.

A 6-year-old's brain already has experienced its most rapid growth and has almost all of the neurons it will have, but even in adolescence, some brain systems are still developing. During childhood, the brain grows larger but doesn't add neurons. Instead, it adds complexity to neurons and changes mental capacities that correlate with developing brain regions, such as increasing self-control.

Scans of children and adolescents show how the brain develops from the back to the front. Regions necessary for sensation, movement, and many basic emotional and sexual responses are fully formed first. Frontal regions necessary for self-restraint, short-term memory, and future planning are not necessarily fully mature in young adults. This physically changing brain results in changing behaviors. Risk-seeking decreases and hazardous behavior declines after the teen years. Children diagnosed with attention deficit disorder often grow out of it as their brains mature.

As growing neocortical neurons send out dendrites, they increase the thickness of the **gray matter**. Although the eventual thickness of the gray matter is similar, the timing of this change is important. Thickening happens later in high-achieving children, suggesting that appropriately timed growth is an important element. In addition to this gain in bulk, a final stage in brain maturation includes adding a sheath of protein and fat to the axons. This protein is called myelin, and it allows the fast coordination of action, helping impulses travel faster. Because the brain develops from the back of the skull to the front, myelination comes last to the prefrontal regions that control executive function, which entails self-control and planning. This process is not complete until people reach their early 20s.

Mental capacities develop on their own and in response to external events. These capacities have a range of trainability, highlighted below:

- IQ is an innate quality that is difficult to train, although problem-solving intelligence can be improved by working on memory.

- Temperament has genetic and environmental components. Surprisingly, peers have more influence on a child's temperament than parents do, although careful nurturing by parents can help to improve a difficult temperament.

- Will power (self-regulation) probably involves plasticity in the neocortex, the brain systems related to executive function. This trait is an early indicator of academic success in later years and can be trained. Self-control can be taught as early as age 3 by elaborate, imaginative play, including intricate games. Some schools use a program called Tools of the Mind to teach preschoolers self-control and restraint.

- Multitasking is a myth because what we really are doing is switching from one cognitively demanding task to another. That switching between tasks causes a delay. Training can minimize this delay, however. Evidence shows that playing complex video games may involve some element of training for multitasking, because such games require planning and switching tasks, two skills that can broaden the bottleneck in brain processing. ■

Important Term

gray matter: Areas where there are collections of neuronal cell bodies.

1. How might complex play cause long-term changes in brain circuits?

2. In the development of a child's temperament, parental influences may matter less than the daily peer and school environment. Why might this be?

Childhood and Adolescence
Lecture 20—Transcript

Welcome back. So far in considering the development of the brain, we've talked about infancy. We've talked about childhood. Now what I'd like to do in this lecture is follow the developing brain past childhood and into young adulthood. This trail, as it turns out, leads us back to early childhood because of evidence linking these two phases of development. Let's focus on young adulthood and adolescence, and then keep in mind that we're going to be coming back full circle.

Nearly all neurons have been born by the age of six and so the brain is mostly done making neurons by that age. However, development continues through adolescence and into young adulthood. Development takes the form not of adding new neurons, but instead, of adding complexity to individual neurons, for instance, dendrites and axons growing, as well as growth in the total number of synapses connections. So the brain is not yet done growing, and in fact, the brain still grows in size.

One principle that emerges as we watch brains develop both in animals and in humans is that there is a tendency for brains to develop from the back to the front, and that starts in the hindbrain and goes all the way to the forebrain. This is true in other animals as well as in us. It's possible to see this development in live action, as it were, by looking at composite images of brains from many different children and young adults, following them over time. It's possible to take brain scans in which one can measure the thickness and the total volume of brain tissue during brain development from childhood to early adulthood. This has been done by a research group that has taken these brain scans from all these many subjects and pseudo-colored it, so pseudo-color is false coloring, and what they've done is visible in this movie here. So now, let's look at this movie.

This is a movie that's a composite movie of human cortical development, the development of the neocortex, from childhood to early adulthood. The darkest colors here, the blue and the purple, denote parts of the cortex that are fully mature. Then the red and green are areas that are not mature yet. The bottom of the image is the occipital pole of the cortex, the back of the brain. The top part is the frontal pole of the brain. So this is showing the front of the brain at the top of the screen, and the back of the brain in the bottom of the screen. What we can see here is that in this composite image over many subjects, many children and young adults, is that the brain develops from back to front. You can see that the brain has largely reached its mature thickness and volume in the back first, and then gradually progresses. You can see the spread on the blue and purple from the back to the front of the brain.

That's interesting because this is a change that's happening in children as they approach young adulthood. What that means is as follows. The change in the brain developing, the maturation of the brain from back to front, means that regions necessary for sensation, movement, and many basic emotional and sexual responses are fully formed first. They're formed before frontal regions, which we've heard about a lot. Those frontal regions are necessary for self-restraint, short-term memory, and making plans for the future. What that means is that those frontal functions might not necessarily be fully mature in young adults.

If that reminds you of anything, then let's think a little bit about adolescents. Adolescents often are reported to not have very good ability to make plans for the future, exercise restraint, or remember things. So it's a possibility that perhaps this developmental progression may form the physical basis for adolescents perhaps having less of these capabilities than they will eventually have when they grow up. So the late development of frontal regions could underlie the improvement in those things that happen after adolescence.

Another example of this may be, for instance, attention deficit disorder. This is a phrase that we've been hearing a lot in the last few years. It is often the case that teens and children are diagnosed with this. But now combine that with the fact that we're now looking at this movie showing brain development. And what that shows is the brain is not developing yet. It turns out that diagnosed attention deficit disorder is often resolved simply by waiting a few years. That perhaps is not surprising given what we've just seen about brain changes that happen throughout development.

There is another principle of brain development. I've just shown you this general principle of the brain developing from back to front. Another principle of brain development is one that fits with a lot of what we've been talking about, about brain plasticity. That's that neocortical neurons, neurons in the brain, in the neocortex can branch and proliferate. I've talked about neurons being born by the age of six. These neurons continue to branch and proliferate. Specifically, neurons send off a dendrite. They send off dendrites in various directions. One dendrite comes out from the neuron's cell body and goes out towards the outer surface of the brain. It starts in the cell body and goes out to the outer surface of the brain. The longest dendrites span the entire thickness of the grey matter of the neocortex. What that means is that as these neurons grow and proliferate in that direction, one would then expect to see increases in the thickness of the grey matter. In fact, it's possible to see these changes in the average, in the bulk, by doing brain scanning and looking at scans of the entire brain like the one we just looked at.

As it turns out, it has been observed that the grey matter of the cerebral cortex, the neocortex, does increase in thickness throughout childhood. It's possible to look at a composite movie in which one can follow this over time. It's possible to see changes in the thickening of the grey matter in children and in adolescents. One finding that is very interesting is that there is a relationship between the thickening of the grey matter and intellectual ability, measured performance on IQ tests. But it's not exactly the change that one might expect. Naively you might expect, I don't know, thicker grey matter, higher IQ, or something like that. That's not exactly what happens. It turns out that the eventual thickness of the grey matter reaches about the same levels in high achieving and non-high achieving children. But what happens is that the thickening is observed to happen relatively later in higher achieving children. So they all reach a similar final thickness, but the thickening happens later in higher-achieving children.

It's not known why that is. It seems odd, perhaps even paradoxical. But what it suggests is the idea that appropriately timed growth is the important thing. There is something about growth that needs to happen at the right time as opposed to indiscriminate growth. The reason for why this would be is not known. I should say at this point, I think we should pause and say that the reasons for it are not known, and also there are variations among individuals. So what that means is that there is no action item for parents. You should not go out and get your kids scanned. You should not go, I don't know, to find an exercise to delay the thickening of the grey matter. There is no finding here that's cause for action. It is simply an observation that suggests that there is something about brain development that you can see in the bulk that is predictive, that correlates with, intellectual development, which is interesting.

There is a final stage in brain maturation. So far I've talked about just simply the addition of bulk and also the branching of dendrites. But there is also a stage of brain maturation that I haven't mentioned before, and it's the addition of a protein called "myelin." Myelin is a material that's made of protein, also of fat. It's a sheath that surrounds axons. It's a sheath that allows fast coordination of activity. The way it allows this is what it does is it ensheath an axon and makes impulses travel more quickly. It also makes them use less energy. So this myelin allows fast coordination of activity throughout the brain because when pathways in the white matter are covered in myelin, then conduction across the brain can be quite fast.

Like the development of brain matter from back to front that I showed you in the movie, myelination also comes last in prefrontal regions. We're back again into the subject of executive function, including planning and self-control. Myelination is not complete until people reach their early 20s. Again, that suggests a possible physical basis for changes in self-control and changes in the ability to pay attention. So there is this sense that one gets from these changes in brain structure, that there is a physical basis in the kinds of capacities that change as we go through adolescence and reach early adulthood.

Let's now back up and talk, once again getting away from the cellular structures of biology of individual cellular components. Let's get back to how mental capacities are a combination of native ability and trainability. Let's talk about how mental capacities develop on their own and also in response to external events. It turns out that mental capacities have a range of trainability. They range from things that are very hard to train, to things that are relatively trainable. I'll give you a few examples of the extremes and then something that is somewhat in between.

One mental capacity that is relatively hard to train by practice is IQ. Recall that I told you before about the role of the first three years of life and the environment that children encounter in those first three years of life on later IQ. That's true, but it is also the case that IQ is a hard thing to train. In fact, IQ tests were originally designed to give an unvarying measure of intelligence. So there is a sense in which IQ is supposed to measure some innate quality, and indeed, it is the case in fully grown adults and also in children that IQ is a relatively hard thing to train. There is some evidence that fluid intelligence, which is problem-solving intelligence, can be trained a little bit by training working memory. But by-and-large, IQ is a hard thing to train.

A more easily trainable capacity is self-control. Recall in the lecture on willpower, I talked about self-control and I talked about things like wrong-handed tooth brushing and doing things that required restraint. I talked about those things like sticking with an exercise program as a means of building one's ability to exert self-control. We're going to come back to this. But that's an example of something that is more trainable.

Then there is a capacity that is somewhat in between, and that is a person's temperament. So the kind of personality that a kid has, say for instance whether a child is very anxious or very calm, those capacities, temperament, are mostly genetic. They are mostly genetic, but at the same time, there is an environmental component. What that means is that there is a certain degree to which a child's temperament is influenced by his or her environment.

We're right on the edge of an action item. You might imagine that the next recommendation would be, well, parents should do something to improve the temperament of their children because they have some influence. But there is something odd, which is that even though there is an environmental influence on temperament, the influence appears not to come from parents. When people have studied this, it has been very hard to find evidence of parental influences on children's temperament. So, what's left? Well, what's left is the peer group. Children spend a lot of time with their peers, and so one possibility is that, in fact, peer groups may, in fact, have some influence on temperament.

There is some evidence that in the extreme, temperaments can be influenced by nurturing from a parent. There is some evidence that, for instance, the most anxious babies and children can benefit from the right kind of nurturing to bring them back from being a very anxious person. So there is some evidence that there is an effect of nurturing. But mostly it's pretty hard to influence a child's temperament. I think that if you've ever had the experience of raising a child, well, if you've ever been a child and been raised, then you know that there is a lot of difficulty in influencing a child's temperament.

Let's take this and put it together a little bit. The lesson that I would like to summarize here at this point is that although the most rapid changes in brains happen before the age of six, growth and maturation continue all the way through adolescence and beyond. These changes rely on programs that are set up by genetics. They are also influenced by the environment. So, at the same time, the developing brain, the changing brain, uses cues from the surrounding world, presented at the right time in development, recall the sensitive period concept, and those cues help the brain help you develop abilities and skills that are matched to the demands of the environment. So that's a capsule summary of what we've learned so far about development.

I want to talk about one kind of mental capacity that can be trained, and I want to put together a few threads that we've been developing over the last lectures. I want to talk about willpower and self-regulation. I want to now talk about this in the context of child development.

Recall that when I talked about willpower, I talked about the marshmallow test as applied to preschoolers and its consequences. Recall that I said that self-control in preschoolers is a predictor of school success. It's a predictor of school success not only that year, but it also predicts academic success years later, during adolescence. It predicts regard by one's peers. This is interesting because self-control is what one might call willpower. In that lecture I talked about how willpower can be taught in adults. It's likely to involve plasticity in the neocortex, in particular brain systems that are involved in the executive attention.

In the last few lectures we've talked about how plastic young brains are and how brains are developing in young people from childhood through early adolescence. So now it's time for the other shoe to drop. The other shoe dropping is as follows. There are recent findings that self-control can be taught as early as the age of three. What this means is that it's possible to teach self-control to children and get them to be better at it. It turns out to not be something that's taught by making a child exert self-control. That's sort of dreary. The way to do it is by imaginative elaborate play, the kind of play that children enjoy, the kind of play that they can, in fact, get very absorbed in. This kind of imaginative elaborate play translates to better academic performance and regard from peers.

I should say that this is not just any kind of play. So, it's a commonplace statement that children should just be allowed to be children and just go play and be free. There are even schools of preschool and early education in which children are felt to just benefit from just running around loose. That turns out not to be the kind of play that's helpful in building up this self-control. The necessary ingredient appears to be mature and dramatic play, intricate games, in which planning and impulse control are involved. For instance, two little girls playing and having a tea party, so having a tea party where you set up the cups. You have the dishes. You say, "Okay, I'm going to pour the tea. You have the tea. You come over to my house," complicated games that require a lot of drama and a lot of planning, and a lot of restraining oneself. These kinds of play are helped by having mediating activities, mediating objects, that can get the kids to hold still and to restrain themselves in ways that they normally would not.

So, here is an example. When children are asked to stand still, a three-year-old, they typically can't make it past one minute. They stand, and they stand, and they stand. And they can't take it anymore, which is sort of marshmallow-test like. But if they play a game in which they pretend to be guards and they're guarding a factory, they can stand at attention for more than four minutes. So there is something about elaborative play that allows children to exert self-control and to do things that help them restrain themselves.

Play can be directed then. In this way, children's ability to control their cognitive acts, to control their actions and their thoughts, can be shaped. For instance, it's possible to say have children make a plan for what they'll do. So you can ask a child, "Well, what I would like you to do today is tell me what your plan is for the day. What are you going to do? Oh, you're going to build a sand castle or you're going to have a tea party? Oh, that's great!" And so let the kid go off and then check in later with the kid and ask her, "Well, did you stick with that plan because, you know, it's time for the tea party now and it's time to have the tea party." And so this idea of complex play is a way in which children can be engaged in an enjoyable way in the process of elaborative play.

And this taps into beliefs that date back to early pioneers in child development and the study of child development by psychologists such as the Russian scientists Alexander Luria and Lev Vygotsky. They had a belief that play was something very serious. They believed that play was an important part of learning how to become adults. Vygotsky had ideas about what play was and what it was important for, and he had thoughts such as the following. He thought that make-believe is more stimulating, more satisfying, and more fun, if you stick to your role. If you have your role and you stick to it, if you're guarding the factory, if you're having the tea party, if that's more fun. He believed that when children followed the rules of make-believe and pushed one another to follow these rules, they're developing important habits of self-control. So play is, in some ways, an activity that doesn't make all that much sense. It's a universal practice in mammals. All mammals play. It seems to be harmless practice for adult activities, but it turns out that in this case, complex play has a useful outcome.

I've set up this idea of complex play being helpful for small children. This has been studied in the specific context of executive function. These are studies that are ongoing that have been done in the last few years. There is a study done by Adele Diamond and her colleagues done a few years ago. What they found is that executive function skills, these things that we've been talking about quite a lot, can be taught to preschoolers as early as the age of three or four. They can even improve school performance more than other preschool programs. This is published in *Science* magazine and it's a program that's called "Tools of the Mind."

Tools of the Mind turns out to be a simple program. It doesn't require special equipment. It doesn't require specially educated people. It only requires training of teachers, and it just requires the preschool teachers to be taught how to engage children in complex play. Teachers usually regard play as unsupervised time, a break from work. But in this case, the right kind of play can be used to get something done. There are examples of these Tools of the Mind.

One example is an example called "Buddy Reading." Buddy Reading is an activity in which children have a mediating object, and the mediating object can be something like a little picture of an ear. You take the picture of the ear and you say, "Okay, now when you are holding the ear, it's your turn to listen." Then the kid holds the ear and listens to the other kid reading the book. Then the other kid is reading the book. Then when the other kid is done reading the book, then the first kid hands her the ear and says, "Okay, now it's your turn to listen. Now it's my turn to talk." If there is a concrete external aid that's used to help activities such as Buddy Reading so that kids know when it's time to behave and know when it's time to talk or not talk. So, that's an example of a tool that's used in Tools of the Mind.

Another example is regulating the behavior of others. So, for instance, maybe one child might have a thing to do which is maybe write down the numbers 1 through 10. Then the other kid would go and check the behavior and say, "Well, did you write down the numbers 1 through 10?" One child might regulate the behavior of others. Some children do this naturally, by the way. There are some children who actually really enjoy it.

Another thing that's taught to children by these teachers is to use private speech, private speech to regulate oneself or to switch roles in a complex task. So, for instance, teachers might encourage the children and say, "Well, why don't you talk about what you're going to do." "Well, I'm going to go over here and I'm going to pour the tea. And I'm pouring the tea, and I'm putting the pot on the stove." So there is a component of using private speech, the children using private speech to regulate themselves or to switch roles when they are doing something complex.

Finally, the thing I talked about before with the tea party, mature, dramatic play. These are the components of this Tools of the Mind program and after some period of practice, it is possible to measure improvements in executive function. What they've done now, what these investigators have done, is they've measured executive function. It turns out that executive function is something that can be measured in a psychology laboratory. What you can do is give a task to children that have difficult and easy parts to them and make them switch. This is a task called "the dots task." It's very closely related to tasks that one could get a monkey to do in the laboratory or human subjects, grown up subjects, in the lab to do.

It goes like this. So, this a task in which the child is asked to look at a fixation point, to look at a plus sign in the middle, and say, "Okay, when you see the heart, well, you should push a button that's on the same side as the heart." That's called "a congruent task" where you push on the same side. Then this is a task that comes very naturally to children. You push the button on the same side. If the heart is on the left, you push on the left. If the heart is on the right, you push on the right. That's an easy task.

There is a harder task that children have some difficulty with and it's what some people call "the anti-task." It goes like this. Okay, there is a flower. Now when you see the flower, if you see the flower on the left, push on the right; if you see the flower on the right, push on the left. You can see that this goes against the natural tendency to push the button on the same side as the thing that shows up. So that's the anti or incongruent task.

The hardest task of all is to mix the two up. So, for instance, if you see a heart, push on the same side. If you see the flower, push on the other side. This mixed condition is hardest. This mixed condition is a test of executive function because it requires switching between the same side rule and the opposite side rule.

It turns out that children who are in regular preschool and children who are part of this Tools of the Mind group have been tested on this dots-mixed task, this execution function task. That task, the mixed-dots task can only be done by 30 percent of the control group, but by over half of the Tools group. So, this test of executive function suggests that there is something that executive function has been trained in these kids, so that they become better at it. So, over half of them can do something that kids who get regular treatment have, in fact, a fair amount of difficulty with.

One thing that's been interesting about this Tools of the Mind Program is that it has been tried out in a number of schools, and there has even been a report in a school in which the administrators at the school see the Tools kids and see the non-Tools kids, and called a halt to the program. The reason that they called a halt to the program is that they say, "Well, the Tools kids are doing much better, and we think it's not fair to deprive the other kids of that. And so, we're just going to call a halt to the study. Everybody has got to get the Tools treatment." So that's a benefit that appears to be noticeable to people who are running the school and they can see in the children a benefit, and they want all the kids to get the benefit.

This benefit translates to increased ability at a variety of academic pursuits. I mentioned that there are these different dots tasks. There is the congruent task, which is the easy one, the incongruent task, which requires going in the opposite direction, and in particular, the mixed-dots task, that's the hardest one in which the children have to switch back and forth between the two tasks. That one is predictive of other scores measured at the end of the year, such as getting ready to read, when the kids are taking tests to see whether they are on the threshold of starting to read, which is something that kids, three-and four-year-olds, are ready for. So what appears to be the case is that executive function predicts ability to succeed at the end of that year. Now what I'm showing you is that it is something that can be trained in children. It's something that can be taught by getting kids to play in complicated and interesting ways.

Recall what I said before which is that executive function is also correlated with school performance. Executive function, as it turns out, in work done by Duckworth and Seligman, shows that executive function is a correlate of school performance even through high school. So what that shows is that this executive function appears to be something, remember I mentioned before, that it's more predictive of academic success than IQ.

Now finally, last example, I want to give you one more kind of training that happens a few years later in childhood. So now we're getting out of the preschool years and we're getting into later childhood. This relates to a phenomenon colloquially multi-tasking. First off, we need to take care of a myth. The myth is the phenomenon of multi-tasking. We often talk about being able to multi-task and being able to do one thing and another thing, being able to have a conversation on the phone and work on a document or whatever it might be that we're doing. We believe that we can multi-task, but it turns out that in a deep sense, true multi-tasking is a myth. Multi-tasking is called by experimenters "task switching." So whenever you switch from one cognitively demanding task to another one, that takes a little bit of time because you need to basically focus your attentional spotlight from one thing to another. What that means is that task switching imposes delays whenever we have more than one task requiring our active attention. So it's possible, for instance, to process multiple sensory motor activities at once. It's possible to walk and chew gum. But focused attention on multiple cognitively challenging tasks is hard. There is a bottleneck in brain processing.

That's the fact about multi-tasking. It's sad but true. It turns out though that there is a certain extent to which it can be reduced. This bottleneck can be broadened a little bit with practice. So even though you can never get the multi-tasking delay, the task switching delay, to go away, you can at least get the delay to be reduced somewhat. In fact, there is evidence that complex video games may have some element of training. It may be possible that training children, when children practice say some complex video game such as Sim City or some other video game involving a lot of planning and complex switching of tasks, that that complex cognitive process can, in fact, reduce the time cost of task switching. Of course, playing video games is something kids these days do a lot of. What this goes to show is that perhaps the right kind of video games, with enough complexity, could in fact be beneficial in a practical, everyday skill.

Let's summarize what we've learned today. Let's back up and back up a little bit of the last lecture, and talk about this lecture. The brain continues to develop through childhood into young adulthood. Young adulthood includes adolescence. Adolescence is a time when some brain systems are fully grown, and others, for instance, prefrontal systems, are still growing. All throughout this time the brain is changing, and along with the brain changing, behavior is changed as well. So for instance, the tendency to seek risks decreases. Hazardous behavior goes down from the teen years to adulthood. But also, problems like attention deficit/hyperactivity disorder, ADHD, tend to go away on their own. These are reflections of the constantly changing brain from childhood through adulthood.

All through this time, the brain can also learn. One capacity that can be practiced in preschoolers is self-control, just as it can be practiced in adults. Self-control in preschool is a predictor of later life success. What this suggests is something interesting and I'll speculate at this point; it may be that early childhood interventions to practice self-control can result in school improvements in the long-term. So that's an exciting possibility that I think will be tested in the coming years.

Now that we've talked about development from childhood through adolescence, in the next lecture what we'll talk about is yet another thing that's a combination of inborn tendencies and environmental influence, and that particular thing is hands dominance.

Handedness—Sports, Speech, and Presidents
Lecture 21

The general theme is that left-handers are more variable than right-handers. They are more likely to get a high SAT score. They are more likely to be more creative. But they are also more likely to be criminals or mentally retarded. So there is this greater variation in left-handedness.

Why is an important assistant called a right-hand man and not a left-hand man? Why do we favor one hand over another, beginning in infancy? Of all the animals, only humans predominantly favor right-handedness. Other species have either no preference or favor one hand for one skill and the other hand for another skill. Only 1 in 10 people favor left-handedness, an attribute with negative cultural myths but one that fascinates neuroscientists, who believe that it arises from a mix of genetic and environmental causes.

Myths about left-handedness include beliefs that left-handers have shorter life spans and are more accident-prone and the idea that right-handedness is just better than left-handedness; these ideas have been debunked. There are no known biological disadvantages for left-handedness.

What is true is that left-handers are more variable than right-handers both in the high and low end of achievement, and they seem to think differently in many ways, ranging from creative arts to SAT scores. There are more lefties in the creative arts (Pablo Picasso was one), and lefties have unusual math skills; dealing with a right-handed world encourages divergent thinking—finding counterintuitive solutions to problems. Interactive sports (baseball, fencing, tennis, and boxing) are dominated by lefties, which may be because left-handers' better-developed right hemispheres give them an advantage. Another explanation is that both right-handed and left-handed athletes have less experience facing a left-handed opponent. Both right-handers and left-handers have more difficulty anticipating a lefty's next move. Lefties are also more likely to be criminals or mentally retarded.

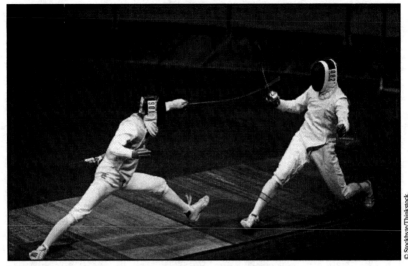

© Stockbyte/Thinkstock.

Interactive sports are dominated by left-handed people.

Neuroscientists have multiple theories on how handedness is determined, including genetic, experience-dependent, and environmental/early developmental models. Early life preference can lead to a cascading effect in which practice leads to eventual dominance of one hand. A brain injury to the brain's left hemisphere, which controls the body's right side, could require a person to compensate and use the left hand. This could account for left-handers' unusually high rate of neurological disorders. Or perhaps a person began with an innate preference but made an early decision to use the left hand.

Six of the past 12 U.S. presidents have been left-handers and noted orators, illustrating the belief that there is some fundamental link between hand dominance and language, which is lateralized, or processed, in both hemispheres. The left side (Broca's and Wernicke's areas) processes inputs and outputs. The right side processes nonverbal, non-language abilities, including prosody, or the melody of speech, its emotional content. Most people process language on the left side of the brain, but a study showed that 10% of left-handers processed language on the right side of the brain; another 15% processed language on both sides—something rare in right-handers. Why is this? Perhaps using the left hand early in life allows both sides of the brain to process language. Maybe verbal and manual dexterity go together because they use common neural structures. ∎

Questions to Consider

1. Do left-handers have shorter life pans than right-handers? What is the problem with the evidence?

2. What is the connection between handedness and language? What evidence does brain imaging provide on this subject?

Handedness—Sports, Speech, and Presidents
Lecture 21—Transcript

Welcome back. In the last few lectures we have talked about development starting from infancy and going through adolescence, ways in which brains change as babies grow up to be young adults.

Today what I would like to do is talk about a specific trait that is one way in which children start to become differentiated from one another in the first few years of life, and that trait is handedness.

What I would like to do today is talk about the biology of where handedness comes from, whether animals have it, implications for brain function, facts and myths about handedness. And finally, I would like to talk about implications that handedness may have for function in our lives and in the lives of public figures that we encounter in the news.

First, let's talk about the question of whether other animals are handed. It is true that other animals do show some hand preference, or in the case of animals, paw or foot preference. So, for example, let us look at rats. Rats do have a paw reference, and so when you give rats a task to do, rats will either use the right paw or the left paw. So that is certainly the case. However, rats don't have a strong preference, left or right. As a group, equal numbers rats prefer the left paw to the right paw.

Crows though, for example, to take a second example, do not have hands, but they do make asymmetric tools. So, for instance, crows will make tools by clipping a branch or a leaf, and then keep that tool for later. So again there is a left/right asymmetry that is recognized by crows. So that is another example in which one can see evidence for handedness or left/right preference in a fairly complex bird, a crow.

To take an example of an animal that is relatively close to us, chimpanzees also have hand preference like us, and they have a hand preference in which they will, in the wild, wild chimpanzees will have a the hand preference for fishing termites out of the nest or for instance for cracking a nut. In that case, even though they showed left-hand or right-hand preference for these different tasks, their handedness is in fact mixed. They will, in fact, prefer the left hand for one task, the right hand for another task.

So one tendency we see in other animals is there is not a real strong feeling for having a strong preference for having left-handedness or right-handedness. In fact, it is often the case that other species are not terribly discriminating in the difference between left and right. So for instance, it is fairly common for nonhuman animals to have trouble distinguishing mirror images from another. So if you show an animal an image like, this or an image like this, they are not necessarily going to be very good at telling that difference.

So that is what we can see in other animals, a handedness, but not a strong preference overall within a species for left or right. What that suggests is that there is something different about us. There is something about left-handedness that is somehow linked closely with our brains, perhaps the complexity of our brains, and I am going to get into that in a moment.

First, what I would like to do is talk about cultural beliefs about left-handedness. These are beliefs that many people hold about left-handedness. As it turns out, many of those beliefs are negative. In fact, the negative beliefs are almost entirely myths. So I will give you a few examples.

For years, left-handedness was an object of suspicion. This goes back for millennia and it shows up in our language. So for instance, a right-hand man is indispensable. If you are a dancer—if you are dancing—and your partner has two left feet then that is a person to be avoided. If you look in the Bible, in the New Testament, sinners who do not meet with the Savior's approval go to his left and they go to eternal damnation.

If you look in the language, if you look at languages around the world, you can see words for left and right that have positive and negative connotations. So for instance, "adroitness" and "dexterity" derive from French and Latin words, respectively for right, whereas "gauche" and "sinister" derive from words for left.

So all of these are examples of cultural beliefs in which it is very clear that there some believe that there something different between left and right.

And, in fact, in most of these cases the belief is that right is somehow superior to left.

In the face of all this perhaps it is no wonder that well into the 20th century in countries around the world, children who showed signs of left-handedness when writing were forced to switch hands. What that means is that at least 1 in 10 people have a natural tendency to be left-handed, and it means that 1 in 10 schoolchildren were forced to switch hands early in life.

This practice has faded in many developed countries. So for instance, in the United States left-handed kids are now allowed to stay left-handed. But it turns out that it is still done in some countries. For example, in modern Japan children are still compelled to use their right hands when they write. So that is something that is still done in schools in Japan.

So those are cultural beliefs about right-handedness, left-handedness and cultural biases. Now I want to specifically address some ideas about left-handers, some of which are even believed by many left-handers. So here is one idea.

Even today, left-handers are thought to be accident prone. This turns out to be a myth. When you look at the rates of accidents between left-handed and right-handed persons, for instance in automobile accidents or machine shop accidents, there is no difference in the rate of accidents despite the fact that automobiles and machine shops, in fact, have handed tools—steering wheels, various machine shop tools, have a certain handedness—yet there is no difference in accident rate.

There is one belief that is quite common; the belief that, in fact, left-handers don't live as long as right-handers. There is a lot of apprehension among many left-handers. In 1991, one US-Canadian research team reported that left-handers died on average nine years earlier than right-handers. What those researchers speculated was well maybe it is because of higher rates of accidents or disease. This came out in the news, and when the story came out in the news, those researchers received a hailstorm of criticism, including death threats. People really got worked up about this finding.

The resulting media attention led to careful examination in that team's methods uncovered, in fact, a fatal flaw. The fatal flaw was one of biased samples. This is always a concern when sampling human populations, because you have to take what you can get when you go to a human population to study some characteristic. You do not have the luxury of, say, going to the laboratory and picking animals and doing something with the animals.

So, here, what they did is they looked in the population for left-handers and right-handers. Recall that I said that for much of the 20th century left-handers were discouraged from using their left hands. What that means is that because left-handers were long discouraged from using their dominant hand. That means that many older people, whose innate tendencies would place in the left-handed population, were scored by researchers in general, as being right-handed. As a result, there are no old left-handers, so these deaths of these people were recorded as right-handed deaths.

In other words the way to think about it is that the reason that these researchers didn't see any old left-handers was that left-handers had all converted to being right-handed. Consequently, they did not see any old left-handed people. They concluded that in fact left-handers did not live as long, but in fact, they just were masquerading as right-handers.

A well known counterexample is US President Ronald Reagan. Ronald Reagan is said to have been left-handed. He used his left hand for many everyday tasks, but he wrote with his right hand. In fact, he lived to the age of 93, so a very long time.

One category in which left-handedness is said to make a difference is in sports. If you look in surveys of athletes at the very highest levels of competition in a number of sports, left-handers are in fact overrepresented. Examples include tennis, fencing, and boxing. All these are sports in which you can see left-handers at well above the natural incidence in the population, which recall I said was about 1 in 10. So more than 1 in 10 left-handers, well more than 1 in 10 left-handers are represented at the top ranks of these sports.

One well-known example is baseball pitchers. Baseball pitchers on a baseball diamond typically face west if you are on a conventional baseball diamond. So they face west to pitch to the batter. When they're left-handed, therefore, their hand is to the south. What that has led to is the slang term "southpaws." So left-handed people are often called "southpaws" and it comes from this phenomenon of baseball pitchers.

That is an example of, again, left-handedness being overrepresented in a particular area of athletic performance. Why is it that left-handers are overrepresented? There are two different kinds of explanations, and one kind of explanation is that there is some kind of neurological advantage in the player, him or herself. It goes like this. The idea is that in most people, the left hemisphere of the brain and the right hemisphere of the brain developed to different extents. The left half the body is controlled by the right half of the brain, and the right half of the brain tends to be somewhat less developed than the left half of the brain. So one suggestion has been, well, if you are left-handed, then you have a better developed right hemisphere and perhaps that gives southpaws some kind of natural advantage. That would be one possibility for why it is that there might be and advantage.

Another possibility is that well, maybe if they are left-handed then perhaps there is better coordination between the hemispheres of the brain. So these are explanations that reside in the brain of the left-hander, him or herself. But there is another category of explanation that has a little bit more to do with the brain of the left-hander's opponent. This more hinges upon the relative rarity of left-handers. I will give you a few pieces of evidence that suggest that it is not necessarily the brain of the left-hander.

The first piece of evidence is that recall the list of sports that I gave you in which left-handers have an advantage. They were all interactive sports—tennis, fencing, boxing, baseball—these are all sports in which you have an opponent who you have to work with or against in order to get an advantage.

It turns out that there is no left-handed advantage observed in noninteractive sports. So I will give you a few. There is no particular preponderance of left-handers in cycling, gymnastics, or swimming. These are sports where left-handers are not overrepresented. Other examples include darts, tenpin bowling, or golf.

One amusing example you find literature is that there is no left-handed advantage in tossing the caber. So it turns out that there is no special advantage to being left-handed when you are tossing the caber, which perhaps is not all that surprising.

So this is a wide range of sports, noninteractive sports for which there is no left-handed advantage. In fact, for some of these sports there is an additional problem, which is that left-handed equipment is often more difficult to get a hold of and so there is a limitation in what clubs or whatever it is that you need for a sport you can get a hold of.

So there is a simple possibility that arises now that I have described— interactive, noninteractive sports. The simple possibility is that left-handers are more rare, and therefore their opponents are less likely to encounter them and therefore have less practice in dealing with a left-hander.

There is a recent study that provides support for this. It is a study of tennis players and goes like this. A group of left-handed and right-handed tennis players were given video clips of tennis strokes to watch. The video clip is of an opponent and a tennis net, and it is a video clip of the person, the opponent, moving towards the ball, and the clips end at the moment that the racket touches the ball. The people watching these clips were asked, could you please predict the direction and depth of where you think the ball is going to land. It turns out that the people watching these clips did better when the opponent was right-handed than when the opponent was left-handed. They were better at predicting where the ball was going to land if the opponent was right-handed.

What is interesting here is that this difference was seen not only when the viewer was right-handed, but also when the viewer was left-handed. So regardless of the handedness of the viewer, both left-handed and right-handed viewers were both better able to predict the outcome of the right-handed opponent versus the left-handed opponent.

So what that suggests is that it is some kind of difference in experience, because the thing that left-handed and right-handed players have in common is they both have more experience with right-handed opponents than with left-handed opponents.

This is interesting from a neuroscientific point of view because there are categories of explanation that this doesn't match. For instance it is possible that perhaps left-handed players might have an easier time imagining the movement of their opponent. It turns out that there are neurons in the brain that are found that fire when we perform an act and also when we see someone else performing the same act.

For instance there would be neurons in my brain that fire when I drink from a glass of water, and if I were to see you drinking from a glass of water then those same neurons would fire. Those neurons are called "mirror neurons." They have been suggested to be a possible mechanism for how left-handers or right-handers can imagine what their opponents are doing. The fact that left-handed and right-handed tennis players have same preference, or same preferred ability, for predicting what right-handed opponents would do suggests that this kind of mirror neuron based explanation cannot account for the advantage held by a left-handed opponent.

Another example is found in cricket, which is played around the world. The advantage here is that left-handed batsmen have an advantage. These left-handed batters do better. They do better against the bowler. So the bowler is a pitcher. So the bowler has less of a disadvantage if he or she has more experience bowling to left-handers. In other words, the advantage the left-handed batters have depends on how much experience the bowler has pitching to people like them.

Finally one last note about left-handed advantages, one argument in favor of the rarity argument is that the left-handed advantage never exceeds 50/50 in any sport. So in other words, as the representation of left-handers goes to 50/50 then you would imagine then the advantage of being left-handed would disappear because your opponents would start to be used to you. That ratio turns out to never reverse.

To summarize, the differences here, at least some of them, are consistent with not an advantage in the brain of the left-hander, but more a disadvantage in his or her opponent. So the idea here is that if you have less practice at something—now you are the opponent—if you have less practice at something then perhaps your brain is less good at it. So it is more a matter of seeing opponents with a certain frequency and knowing whether you are accustomed to finding someone who is left-handed or right-handed on the other side of the net or the other side of the boxing ring.

Now I want to turn to things that are relevant for the rest of us who are not professional athletes. I want to specifically talk about brain function of left-handers. I want to specifically address the question of whether there is something in the thought processes of left-handers that are different, whether left-handers think differently. So let's look at some statistics and some findings, both historical findings also test findings.

So one finding is that left-handers and right-handers have the same average SAT scores, the Scholastic Aptitude Test, which is used for college admissions in the United States. Left- and right-handers have the same average SAT scores, but they are overrepresented among the very highest score.

If you look at the very high end of the distribution, left-handers are overrepresented. It turns out that left-handers are also overrepresented at the low end of the spectrum. So there, in fact, is more variation in left-handers. So that is how the average comes out to be the same.

The benefits are not only academic. You can also find an increased incidence of left-handedness in creative arts. Famous examples of people who are very creative who are left-handed include Pablo Picasso and Benjamin Franklin. Left-handers are common among artists and great political thinkers and so one can see this looking over history. Also one can see this looking in surveys of working artists.

Many left-handers also have unusual mathematical skills. It turns out that when you give problems for left-handers to solve, or math problems to solve, left-handers more frequently engage in what is called "divergent thinking."

Divergent thinking is defined as finding an unexpected or counterintuitive solution to a problem, a solution that right-handers would not come up with.

These are all ways in which left-handers seem to differ on average from right-handers. As I said, left-handers vary in other ways. Left-handers also are more common among criminals and the mentally retarded. So in fact, left-handers seem to be more variable. There is a general theme here. The general theme is that left-handers are more variable than right-handers. They are more likely to get a high SAT score. They are more likely to be more creative. But they are also more likely to be criminals or mentally retarded. So there is this greater variation in left-handedness.

This raises the question of where left-handers come from. So if we look, biologically we can ask the question: This variable population, where do they come from? It turns out that theories, hypotheses, of where handedness comes from rely on a variety mechanisms, and different kinds of mechanisms may lead to different outcomes. So the kinds of mechanisms that have been discussed for where handedness comes from fall to the following categories: genetic models for how handedness arises, experience-dependent models, and finally environment and early development. So these are all ways in which handedness can be determined.

There is evidence for a genetic component. So for example, if you look at twins, you can find evidence for this. Twins are always a good place to look for genetic evidence. For example, if you take human identical twins, if one twin is left-handed then the other twin is highly likely to be left-handed as well. So there is a high incidence of co-handedness in twins. This turns out to be true for chimpanzees as well. If you look at identical twin chimps, again there is a tendency for shared preference, say, in fishing the termites out of the nest, that kind of thing.

The other type of explanation is one in which perhaps there is some early life preference that can be genetic, but it can also be environmental. That early life preference then can lead to a cascading effect in which practice then leads to eventual use of that hand.

Finally another category is in early developmental defects. So perhaps there is some problem that happens. So let me describe in detail some of these various routes by which left-handers can arrive at their orientation.

One category is pathological, and if you look at this group, the possibility is that these are people who would have become right-handed, but early in development the suffered some injury to the left side of the brain, the side that controls the right side of the body. So in these people they are not well able to use the left side of their brain. So they compensate by using the intact side of the brain, the right side, and this accounts for perhaps the observation that southpaws have an unusually high rate of neurological disorders. So you would expect, in fact, such a thing to happen because of a pathological mechanism.

Another category, a second group, is people whose brain development occurs normally. In these people everything is fine, and there is in fact an asymmetry that occurs during brain development in most people, except that their brain functions are reversed. So the idea here is that all their brain functions are reversed. So on the left-hand side of the brain we would have language; on the right side of the brain, we would have perceptual capabilities.

These people would express handedness and other left-brain functions that are typical, such as language, in the right hemisphere. It has been shown in imaging studies, in functional MRI studies, that about 1 in 10 left-handers falls into this category. It may be that there is nothing remarkable about their brains except that somewhere in development there was a choice made, there is a path that was altered in which everything was mirror reverse. So that would be an example of just simple mirror reversal.

The third category is special. The third category may be related to this overrepresentation of left-handers in high-performing people. The third category is people whose innate language capacity and handedness are the same as the general population. In other words, their language capacity and handedness are both initially localized to the left hemisphere, the usual arrangement for nearly all right-handers.

But then early in life, they make a decision. Something happens and they begin to use the left hand more often than the right. That early decision then would cascade throughout life to eventually lead to left hand use.

As I said left-handers left-handers and right-handers are no different in academic achievements and other performance indicators on average. But there is a subpopulation of left-handers who perform exceptionally well. It is possible that these standouts have something different, in particular, if they are learned left-handers.

I have started talking about left-handedness and language, and this observation that both language and handedness seem to be co-represented is a key fact that suggests that there is some deep connection. So there is this perhaps unexpected linkage between handedness and language.

I have already mentioned that control of the limbs is crossed so that the left side of the neocortex controls the right hand and the right side of the neocortex controls the left hand. What that means is that in 90 percent of people, the left side of the brain, 90 percent of people who are right-handed, the left side of the brain controls the dominant hand.

But it also turns out that language is lateralized. So in most people language is lateralized, and in particular, what we have are areas that are discovered by neurologists over 100 years ago, Broca's and Wernicke's areas on one side of the brain are areas for generating and comprehending the content of speech. These areas are usually found on the left side of the brain in Broca's and Wernicke's areas.

On the other side of the brain are non-verbal, non-language related abilities. They include for instance prosody. Prosody is what neurologists call an affect of prosody, and that is the melody of speech, the rhythm and intonation, the colors, the emotional content of speech. So if I say, "That's nice." Or if I say, "Oh, that's nice," That would be an example of affect of prosody.

It turns out that the right side of the brain, the other side of the brain, contains a number of nonverbal perceptual capacities, so not just prosody, but other things that are not language related. What that suggests is this asymmetry comes in part from the fact that perhaps one way to think about it is that language is a real hog when it comes to brain space. So language occupies one side of the brain, and then we can find all kinds of other non-language capabilities taking up a corresponding amount of space.

In nearly all persons language processing, Broca's area and Wernicke's areas, in nearly all persons is on the left side of the brain, and that is true for most people. But the story with left-handers is often quite different. If you look in the brains of left-handed people, you can see differences.

There is one study that showed that in right-handers processing is strongly lateralized when performing a language task compared with an auditory attention task. So the idea here is that in fMRI studies you have to compare the thing that you are interested in with some neutral task. This task in this particular experiment, the neutral task was some auditory attention task, one that did not require language.

What the study showed was that in left-handers about 10 percent of them showed preferential language processing on the other side. Instead of showing it on the left side of the brain, it showed it on the right side of the brain. Another 15 percent showed processing on both sides, and that is really interesting, because both-sided language processing is, in fact, quite uncommon in right-handers. So it is 15 percent of left-handers, but it is much less common more, like 5 percent of right-handers.

So there seems to be some difference in the ability to use both sides of the brain and the setup of the brain to use both sides to process language in left-handers than in right-handers. So that is interesting. So why is that? An attractive possibility is that using the left hand early in life may somehow allow both sides of the brain to process language. So this is where the idea comes from that somehow handedness and language may in some ways be closely related to one another in terms of brain mechanisms.

So it could be that using the left hand early in life sets up conditions to allow both sides of the brain to handle language as well as manual manipulations. This balanced arrangement might, for instance, provide more brain space for language. So, in fact, this both-sided brain language processing could account for why left-handers are overrepresented among high scorers on the Scholastic Aptitude Test.

So there is a deep idea here. The deep idea here is that there is some link, some fundamental link, between hand dominance and language. These two capacities seem very different from another, but yet, they seem to co-vary to some extent. What that suggests is that these two capacities share some cause, some cause that leads to lateralization.

Here is one possibility. One possibility is that larger brains, in general, not only in our species, but also other species, seem to show lateralization. Functions start to get concentrated on one side of the brain. One possibility is that it costs a lot of wire. Recall that neurons put out axons. These axons are the wires over which long-distance, and also some short-distance, communication is possible.

So these axons have to be quite long to build a connection all the way across the brain. There might be evolutionary pressure to concentrate functions on one side because if you could concentrate function on one side, then you need less wire to build a long distance circuit. So that is one possibility.

Another possibility is brain plasticity mechanisms. Recall that I have talked repeatedly about this Hebb principle, the idea that cells that fire together wire together. So it could be that activity dependent mechanisms can help maintain a specific function in a small part of the brain, so that when neurons work together they tend wire together. That is a phenomenon that would tend to cause specific areas, such Broca's area or Wernicke's area, to be on one side of the brain.

So the idea here would be that plasticity mechanisms would tend to collect functions that are very, let's say computationally, in a metaphorical sense, computationally intensive, to start occupying smaller spaces so that communication is more efficient.

So why is it then that language and hand dominance go together? Well it is not known, but it seems like, based on the evidence that I have given you, that there is some common developmental cause, whether it be genetic or environmental. There is something fundamentally shared between determining the order of words and determining the details of fine gestures.

In other words, it may be that verbal dexterity and manual dexterity could, in fact, go together because they use common neural structures. Let's think about these both-sided brain types. They are an interesting case. The people who use both sides of the brain might have other advantages. I have talked about the representation of high SAT scores. That is an example of an advantage. There is a special population of people who have to use language a lot, and they are overrepresented with left-handers, just as with tennis players and baseball players and so on.

That population is Presidents of the United States. It turns out that there are a number of prominent left-handed Presidents, and the recent ones that I will name include Ronald Reagan, Bill Clinton, and Barack Obama. All of these men are left-handed.

It turns out if you go back a little bit, since the end of World War II in 1945, 6 out of 12 Presidents have been left-handed, and they are Truman, Ford, Reagan, the first President Bush, Clinton, and Obama. That seems like a lot, and it is. It turns out that as I have said only 1 in 10 people in the general population is left-handed. So having 6 Presidents out of 12 is quite a lot.

It is even the case that in several years, having a left-handed President was basically a foregone conclusion. For example, in the 2008 election, Barack Obama and John McCain were both left-handed. In 1992 there were three left-handed major candidates for President, and they were George H. W. Bush, Bill Clinton, and Ross Perot. When they debated on the same stage, they all wrote notes with their left hands, which is quite a sight. You might have thought that if you watched that debate you might have thought that maybe your screen was reversed.

Given the unusual capacities of left-handers' brains that I have talked about, could it be that there is something about those unusual capacities that shows up in these people? So I mentioned several examples, there are people who are legendary for their ability to speak and communicate, specifically Obama, Reagan, and Clinton. It could be that these three Presidents may have their handedness in part to thank for their gift. So it is perhaps not surprising that left-handers are overrepresented in one of the fiercest competitions of all, namely the race for the White House.

You notice that I have only talked about Presidents since 1945. Why is it that they have only started popping up in the last 50 years? As I mentioned it may be that in fact there were natural left-handers beforehand, but before that the Presidents, in fact, did not overcome the pressure to be right-handed.

If we look at another population, British Prime Ministers, among British Prime Ministers, of which there are 51, there are only two reported left-handers out of 51 British Prime Ministers. The only known left-handed US President before the 20th century was James Garfield. Garfield was ambidextrous. He could simultaneously write the same sentence in Latin with one hand and in Greek with the other hand. He could write in two languages, two classical languages, at the same time. I think that would be an example of exceptional language ability.

Clearly this is not a universal tendency among left-handers, so if I ask you now to think about the first President Bush. He was left-handed but he was, in fact, made fun of by his friends and political opponents alike for the liberties he took with English language.

Now let's summarize what we have learned today about left-handedness. I have told you about hand dominance and I have told you about how hand dominance arises from a mix of genetic and environmental causes, and that laterality in general is widely found among animals. But it is only in humans that right-handedness has taken such a dominant role.

In humans, right-handedness is prevalent. The left side of the brain controls the right hand, which is dominant. But despite popular belief there are no known biological disadvantages for being left-handed.

While there are no known biological disadvantages, it is true that left-handers are more variable than right-handers, both at the high end and the low end of achievement. They really do seem to think differently in many ways, ranging from creative arts to SAT tests.

Language in most people shares the same brain-sidedness as hand dominance. Again left-handers are more variable, but one of the ways in which they vary is both-sided language processing.

The take home advice from all this, then, is if you have a small child or a grandchild, if you see a child starting to use his or her left hand, do not worry about it. You might even have a future artist, scientist, or President on your hands.

In the next lecture what we will do is we will talk about adulthood and aging.

Reaching the Top of the Mountain—Aging
Lecture 22

So what we have here is evidence that in the most fundamental sense, the adult brain can change throughout life by making new neurons. This process of neurogenesis is variable—it can be regulated by experience—and so, in fact, it can be different from person to person, different from animal to animal, depending on circumstances.

Whether we're able to do it gracefully or not, aging is a process that sees some of our functions decline—beginning as early as our 30s—but sees other capacities remain and even improve. This process reflects the principle that the brain changes throughout life, even making neurons long past the time when such development was commonly thought possible.

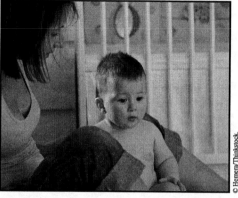

Parenting can encourage neuron generation.

In normal aging, we see structural changes in the brain, as well as behavioral changes in everyday life. Aging brings shrinkage in brain volume and changes in synaptic strength, both with the birth of a few neurons and the loss of others, and changes in dendritic branching and synapses, where the brain actions are carried out. Loss of branching is part of what's responsible for decline in functions, such as memory. Loss of branching may be reversible, but it's harder to replace lost neurons.

The capacity for memory peaks in our 30s, then begins to decline; other functions that decline later in aging are spatial navigation, a capacity shared with some forms of memory, and executive function. This last function

56

includes working memory (what was my friend's phone number again?), speed of response, pattern comparison, processing speed, and self-control. These capacities begin to decline in our 70s and 80s.

It's not all bad news, however. Adult neurogenesis, discovered in 1962 by Joseph Altman, means that the brain (specifically, the hippocampus and olfactory bulb) continues to make a few neurons as we age. And the brain's structural plasticity—its ability to change its structure on the cellular level in response to external events—means that we can have some influence on its natural decline. Stress and **depression** hasten the death of neurons, but active parenting (for both mothers and fathers) and exercise can encourage neuron generation and synaptic strength.

Some functions remain largely unchanged as we age, while others even improve. We generally retain well-learned skills, such as the ability to ride a bike, professional skills, and vocabulary and factual knowledge. (The information is still there, but anomic aphasia, or the Library of Congress effect, will make us slower in recalling it.) Our emotional control improves with age. Our emotional responses become better modulated, and the overall balance tilts toward positive emotion in our 70s and 80s. Neuroscientists suggest two reasons for this functional retention: We have a way to build multiple strategies for solving problems, and we have a cognitive reserve capacity to compensate for neuronal loss.

Unnatural changes that can afflict us as we age include **dementia**, such as Alzheimer's disease; **stroke**; and Parkinson's, which we discussed in an earlier lecture. Alzheimer's is a growing problem as life spans increase, with its likelihood statistically doubling every five years after age 55. Strokes, depriving the brain of oxygen and glucose, are caused by clots or a burst blood vessel. If treated with a specific drug within the first three hours, damage from a clot-induced stroke can be repaired. ∎

dementia: A progressive mental deterioration.

depression: A disorder of "mood" characterized by an internal subjective state of hopelessness and despair.

stroke: Any acute neurological event related to impairment in blood flow or circulation in the central nervous system; can be hemorrhagic or ischemic.

Questions to Consider

1. What capacities decline with age? What capacities stay the same or improve?

2. You think that someone may be having a stroke. How much time do you have to get to a hospital for rapid treatment? Where is the nearest hospital to you that has the appropriate resources?

Reaching the Top of the Mountain—Aging
Lecture 22—Transcript

Welcome back. In the last few lectures we have talked about development, infancy through adolescence, and changes that happen in the brain ranging from infant learning to the development of handedness, to adolescence. In all of these cases these are changes that happened relatively early in life, including childhood and young adulthood. But it is important to remember that that is not the end of the line. The brain is changing throughout life.

So what that means is that the brain continues to change not only as we exit adolescence into young adulthood, but also throughout adulthood and as we get older as well, into old age. What I want to do today is talk about some of these changes that continue throughout life including in the adult brain.

Let's just consider the adult brain in normal adults. As I have mentioned before, synapses can change in strength and that is the phenomena of synaptic plasticity, connections getting stronger or weaker. But there are other changes that also continue throughout life. Even though the great majority of neurons are made by birth, in fact, new neurons continue to be made after birth and throughout life.

So for instance it is the case that the adult brain makes new neurons. This contradicts a large body of evidence going back, and also contradicts a long-standing belief that our brains are done making neurons at an early age. In fact, the idea that our brains do not make new neurons was the prevailing view for over 100 years.

It turns out that this dogma fell about 40 or 50 years ago due to the work, in part, of a biologist named Joseph Altman. Altman, who was forgotten for a while—his work was neglected—used a technique to allow him to visualize new cells being born. This technique of visualizing new neurons being born allowed him to reach the conclusion that, in fact, brains made new neurons.

But as I said, this went against dogma, long-standing, all the way going back into the 19th century. In fact it was the belief that the brain did not make new neurons.

Now it turns out that Altman's findings were not initially accepted. They were in the highest profile journals. They were very well read, but there was something about the idea that was so contrary to existing dogma that they were, in fact, forgotten.

It took decades for the phenomenon of adult neurogenesis, the birth of neurons in new brains, to be rediscovered, and it was rediscovered in birds and also mammals. It was rediscovered using better and better methods. One of the early methods was using a radioactive component of DNA called "thymidine," and if you put radioactive thymidine into tissue, it would get taken up by cells whose DNA was dividing. So cells that were dividing and then subsequently identified to be neurons are, in fact, evidence of newly generated neurons.

There have been subsequent generations of stains, what biologists call ways of labeling tissue. Those are called "stains." These different kinds of stains allow us to identify that a cell is recently generated. And if you put on another stain that is specific to tell you that it is a neuron, that double staining then tells you that, in fact, the new cells that you are observing are neurons.

By now the principle that adult brains can make new neurons at a low rate is by now a well-defined principle. In fact there are several brain regions that generate neurons in the adult brain. One region is the hippocampus, which we have heard about several times. The hippocampus, of course, is important, since it is involved in storing new memories, including facts and events, and also in spatial navigation.

It turns out that one particular part of the hippocampus, the dentate gyrus, is a region that is making new neurons throughout life. Another brain region that makes new neurons is the olfactory bulb. One of the early stages in processing olfactory information, that structure, again, makes new neurons.

It turns out to even be the case that there is some evidence for new neurons being made in the neocortex, the larger part of the brain, the largest part of our brains. In this case the number of neurons that are made in adult brains is quite small. It is a very small trickle. In fact the number is so small that this finding is somewhat controversial. But as far as one can tell from surveying the literature, it appears that the number of new neurons made in the neocortex is not zero, but in fact is some small number.

So what we have here is evidence that in the most fundamental sense, the adult brain can change throughout life by making new neurons. This process of neurogenesis is variable, it can be regulated by experience. And so, in fact, it can be different from person to person, different from animal to animal, depending on circumstances.

I mentioned before the phenomenon of stress in which stress shuts down nonessential biological processes. It turns out that neurogenesis is slowed down in people who are under stress. It is slowed down in lab animals who are under stress. It is also increased in lab animals who are exposed to conditions of environmental enrichment compared with their typical circumstances, and also lab animals that are given the opportunity to exercise. So it appears that neurogenesis is a process that happens in adult brains that can be regulated.

These mechanisms of plasticity are quite potentially important for our lives. So I will give you some examples of findings that come from rodent, monkey, and in some cases, human work. For instance, there is evidence that neurogenesis is reduced in people who are depressed. Treatments that alleviate depression—and now this largely done in animals—treatments that alleviate depression, such as antidepressant drugs, including Prozac, seem to restore neurogenesis. So it is possible to, in fact, chemically restore the phenomenon of neurogenesis with treatments that are also known to alleviate depression.

Another example is social interaction. I mentioned before that stress is something that can affect the brain both when experienced acutely and also chronically. So for instance, when a rat is stuck in a cage with a dominant rat for as briefly as even just a few hours, just a few hours of exposure to a dominant rat can, in fact, affect neurogenesis in a negative direction. So subordination can affect neurogenesis, can suppress it. Likewise chronic subordination can also lead to a reduced neurogenesis.

This is a case in which not only does this manipulation lead to changes in how many new neurons are born, but also changes in structural plasticity.

This brings me to a broader point which is that neurons can change in their structure throughout life, to a certain extent. There is a certain degree to which dendrites can change.

There is a general point which is that many life events, whether stress or other life experiences, many life events can affect both neurogenesis and structural plasticity. So it appears to be the case that the brain can change in its structure, at least at the cellular level, in response to external events, both in the generation of new neurons and also in structural plasticity.

This dual capacity for change means that there are two possible ways in which these kinds of change can affect brain function. So for example, it has been found that at least some new neurons are incorporated into the circuitry of the brain, and there is some question about the permanence of this incorporation. But at least some new neurons are incorporated into the circuitry of the brain.

So these new neurons, even though on average they are small in number, these new neurons are concentrated in some brain regions more than others, concentrated in the dentate gyrus and the olfactory bulb, and may participate in learning and memory. So that is one way in which these phenomena can change the brain.

A second way is structural plasticity; changes in dendrites may be important in influencing brain function. Many of the ways that I have talked about here, I have just mentioned, are ways in which plasticity can be negatively affected by experience. But in fact, there are also ways in which experience can positively affect brain function. So, for example, the act of parenting has been shown to increase dendritic plasticity. It is possible to see increases in dendritic spine density. Those are the little nubs that are in dendrites where the inputs come in. These are changed. For example, it has been demonstrated in marmoset monkeys that the act of parenting can cause growth of dendrites and of spines in the prefrontal cortex. This is specifically in the prefrontal cortex and not in other parts of the cortex, for instance, such as the visual cortex. This is true not only in mothers, as you might expect, but it has actually been specifically observed in fathers. So it is the act of parenting not, for instance, biological gestation. There is something about the act of parenting as a father that affects brain structure.

So the key point that I like to make here to sum up this part is that the brain changes that happened in adult life happen throughout life, not just synaptic plasticity, but also structural plasticity, and in some brain regions, even the generation of new neurons. So this is one principle of change in the adult brain, that is now appreciated and it was not appreciated as recently as a few decades ago.

Now I would like to turn from adult life to things that start happening to our brains and to our capacities as we get older. So what I would like to do is talk about capacities that decline, and in some cases increase, with normal aging. So now let's turn to that.

The general observation is that many of our mental functions are still developing as we go through our 20s. But they also start peaking and then in some cases declining relatively early. For example one capacity that peaks surprisingly early in life is memory, and that includes both long-term memory and also working memory, these two kinds of memory where we recall a fact from long ago or something, some piece of information like somebody's name; but also working memory, when we just try to remember a phone number or some piece of information that we have to look up and then use, like a house number, when you are going to a party, that kind of thing.

These kinds of memory peak around the age of 30, and then decline slowly in most people. So those are forms of memory that decline—forms of mental capacity that decline relatively early, surprisingly early in life.

Another example is spatial navigation. This is interesting because spatial navigation is some capacity that is shared with some forms of memory, namely it involves the hippocampus. And it turns out that one can see in persons starting around the age of 30, one can see hippocampal shrinkage, and the shrinkage in hippocampal volume correlates in time course with loss of function. In the case of rats, what one can see is that the shrinkage in hippocampus also is accompanied by a decrease in dendritic branching.

63

So these are samples of capacities that start to decline relatively early in life, and decline very slowly, gradually, but unmistakably start declining around the age of 30.

Other capacities decline much later, and in these cases the decline happens in a variable way, some people decline later than others and so there is variation among people. But another category of mental capacity that seems to decline is something called "executive function." We have talked about executive function before and we will talk about it in the future. Executive function includes things such as working memory. It includes speed of response. It includes directing one's attention and self-control from task to task. It also includes things like processing speed. All of these functions seem to decline, but they decline later, typically starting in the 70s or in the 80s. So these are things that happen to us relatively late in life.

One can ask the question, are there structural correlates, are there things that we can see in the brain that are changing in correlation with these declines in function as we get very old? Generally speaking, it is not a loss of neurons. For instance, if you look in brain tissue in people as they get older, what is not seen is a loss of neurons, that is not the case.

If you look in animals, what you can see is a loss of synapses. If you look animals and also in humans, what you can see is shrinkage in the prefrontal cortex. Again, a shrinkage in brain volume in humans that has a similar time course as loss of function. And in the case of rats, again, a decrease in dendritic branching in these regions.

So this decrease in dendritic branching is extremely important because branching and connections—the connections between neurons, synapses—impinge upon dendrites. Those synaptic connections are where the brains actions are carried out. So what is going on here is that there are changes in branching as opposed to a loss of neurons. These changes in branching, the shrinkage of dendritic arbors, is probably a part of what is responsible for these lost functions. This is important because one can more easily imagine loss of branching being reversible, whereas lost neurons are of course very hard to make up.

One can even find correlations from individual to individual. I mentioned that the individuals vary in the amount of memory loss and vary in the amount of executive function loss. One can find variations among people in their changes in their brain structure as they get older, and this turns out to also correlate with memory loss.

For example, lesions in the white matter are visible in brain scans, and it is possible to see lesions in white matter, shrinkage in white matter, or changes in the white matter, and those changes in white matter correlate with loss of memory in older adults. So the most severe lesions in white matter are correlated with the most severe loss of memory. So this is an example in which one can see losses of brain tissue or shrinkage in brain tissue that correlates with changes in function as we get older.

It turns out that this is not all bad news; not all functions diminish in aging. There are some functions that do not diminish, and in a few cases functions that seem to, in fact, get better.

For example, physical skills, skills that you learn thoroughly when you are young are spared in aging, whether it be riding a bicycle or a tennis stroke. There are certain skills that seem to be retained as we get older.

Another example is professional skills. So for example, if you are a lawyer or doctor or some other kind of expert, a scientist perhaps, there are professional skills that if you practice them a lot, tend to be retained. So there is a tendency for well-learned skills to be retained as we get older.

There is a general observation here which is that anything you learn thoroughly when you are young is likely to be spared as you get older. What that suggests is that there is a way to build up, say, multiple strategies for solving a problem, multiple strategies for solving a task.

Another possibility is that there is some kind of reserve capacity. In other words, once we have learned how to do something, there may be some cognitive reserve, excess capacity that allows us to maintain function as we get older, even in the face of say some amount of deterioration of single neuron-level function.

So this idea of cognitive reserve is one that is very important and it is one that we are going to come back to as we come back to the question of how one can influence the brain and prevent some of these aging-related declines.

Changes in brain function over life follow a pattern. Some things go down, some things plateau, and some things even decrease. So, for instance, I talked about memory and other executive-type functions. Some things that really notably seem to change over life include speed of processing and this includes things like pattern comparisons, letter comparisons, digit-symbol distinctions, identifying the difference between a digit and a symbol.

Another example is working memory. I talked about working memory being lost. Working memory is something that declines with age; long-term memory as well. But other things don't. So, for instance, verbal knowledge and comprehension do not decrease with age. In fact, there is evidence, good evidence, that vocabulary and factual knowledge increase with age and that increase is sustained into the 80s. That is an example of something that is the same or even better as we get older.

Another example is emotional control. This is an area in which older people have a definite advantage. In general, the frequency of negative emotion declines as we get older, until the age of 60, and then levels off. The frequency of positive emotion stays about the same. But what that means is that the balance between positive and negative tilts towards the positive as we get older, until the age of about 60. So we are less likely to perceive negative events and we are also less likely to remember them. In addition, all these negative moods pass more quickly, we are less likely to indulge in name-calling or other destructive behavior when we get upset. So in short, our emotional responses are better modulated and tend towards the positive as we get older. This is an area in which older people very definitely have the advantage.

In addition to these functional changes, it is possible to look at brain scans and see changes in patterns of brain activity as people get older. So, for example, it is possible see changes in the pattern of brain activation during a task. If you look at older adults versus younger adults, older adults show more activation in the frontal parts of the brain and activation across multiple regions of the brain when they are doing the same task compared with young adults. That could be, for instance, as I was saying before, about well-learned skills, it may be that older adults have compensatory strategies for handling some mental task when they are faced with a problem to solve. It may be that learned skills that are well-learned may call upon multiple brain regions. So there is good evidence that patterns of brain activity are different in the old compared with the young, even when they are solving the same problem.

In addition to these natural changes in our brain's activity as we get older, both in our behavior and also in patterns of brain activity as visible on scans, one can also see changes that are not normal. So in addition to normal aging, there are also pathologies. These pathologies are problems that come with aging. These problems are increasingly common as we live longer. As we make it to older and older ages, these become increasingly important problems that afflict us and those that we love.

Most prominently, one example is Alzheimer's disease. Alzheimer's disease is not the same as regular aging. Alzheimer's disease is a disorder in which we are unable to recall key details of our past. It even becomes possible to lose the ability to recognize one's friends and family.

These are serious, debilitating changes. These are upsetting changes in which the person that you know is somehow lost to you. What is seen in the brains of Alzheimer's patients is that the patterns of brain deterioration are different from normal loss.

So far I have talked about normal aging, and normal aging predominately seems to be caused in its earlier stages by changes in executive function, especially memory, and in frontal and striatal regions of the brain. This is a slowly progressing change in the brain that can lead to mild cognitive decline, but also as we get very old, quite often to dementia.

That is as opposed to Alzheimer's disease in which different brain regions are affected first. In Alzheimer's disease, the earliest targets of change are with the medial temporal cortical systems and the associated regions around that. So remember we have talked about the memory system that includes hippocampus and the medial temporal systems. Those regions seem to be affected first in Alzheimer's disease.

It is possible to see these changes when we look in the area of say structures and brain scans. It is possible to look in the area, say for instance, in the frontal regions such as the anterior callosum, it is possible see changes in brain size, in region size, as we get older. Those changes seem to happen in normal aging as opposed to these other changes associated with Alzheimer's disease, which as I said, seem to focus around the medial temporal system, including hippocampus. So it is possible see distinctive patterns of brain change as people get older, in normal aging and also in pathologies such as Alzheimer's disease.

At the cellular level, it is also possible to see changes. So until recently, the definitive way to diagnose Alzheimer's disease was to look at brain tissue after death. What is characteristically seen after death is plaques and tangles; so tangles of protein, plaques of protein, typically surrounding dead cells. These dead cells are neurons, and what is seen in Alzheimer's patients are these plaques and tangles that can be visualized only in histological section.

In recent years it has started to be possible to visualize some of these changes in living persons. In fact there is now a stain of a compound called "Pittsburgh compound B," "PiB," and this turns out to be a compound that you give to a live person and then put them in the scanner. The compound is visualizable and can be seen in parts of the brain of people with Alzheimer's disease. And you see, again, this characteristic concentration of this of plaque staining protein in the medial and temporal regions of brains of people with Alzheimer's disease.

Alzheimer's disease, as I said, is a disorder that is increasing in incidence as our life expectancy gets longer. And in fact, it is a disordered whose likelihood doubles every five years after age 60. So Alzheimer's disease starts out with a very low incidence around 1 percent, and then rises to 50 percent at age 90. In fact, statistically, you can project the likelihood of Alzheimer's-related dementia and demonstrate that if we all live to 100 years of age 3 out of 4 of us, 75 percent of us, would have Alzheimer's disease.

So this is very clearly a problem that even if it does not affect you, may affect someone you love, may affect someone you know. As we live longer, it's increasingly a societal problem that is the subject of great research.

Alzheimer's disease has some genetic component. So there is something known about the genetics of Alzheimer's disease. There are about a dozen susceptibility genes, the biggest one is ApoE 4, which is a gene that accounts for over half of the risk of Alzheimer's disease. It turns out that if you have two bad copies of this gene, the onset of Alzheimer's disease can be much earlier, 15 years earlier. It is not really known why that is.

Let's talk about another form of pathology that happens in older persons, a risk that increases as we get older, and that risk is of stroke. Stroke is an event which consists of deprivation of blood supply, and therefore loss of glucose and oxygen to the brain. Recall that the brain uses a lot of energy, and so deprivation of blood supply is a critical and sometimes catastrophic event in one's life.

Strokes can be caused by multiple causes. One major type of stroke is a clotting stroke. A stroke that starts with a clot of blood, either in the periphery or in the brain itself, and this clot can block blood flow.

Another type of stroke is a bleeding stroke, a hemorrhagic stroke, in which a blood vessel in the brain ruptures and then causes bleeding, and then therefore causes deprivation of oxygen and glucose to some region in the brain.

Stroke is a serious problem. The lifetime risk of stroke among people over age 55 in the United States is 1 in 5. It is somewhat higher in women. Something like 700,000 people last year in the United States suffered a stroke. There about 5 million survivors of stroke today in the United States.

So stroke is a very important disorder, and it is very important to understand at least a little bit about stroke because it can happen to you or to someone you care about quickly and in your presence. There are things that can be done.

Because of the necessity of oxygen and glucose to brain function, damage caused by stroke can begin in just a few minutes. There is some preservation of function that is possible if stroke is caught quickly. So stroke symptoms initially begin as a loss of sensation on one side or loss of ability to move on one side. These are the early signs of stroke, perhaps confusion.

It is possible to preserve some function in the case of strokes that begin with a blood clot. The way this is done is with a drug called "tissue plasminogen activator," which also goes by the name of "alteplase." Alteplase is a drug that when given soon enough can undo the damage caused by a clot. The critical factor here is that you need to get to an emergency room with a PET scanner which allows identification of what type of stroke you are having, because of course the clot-busting drug would be of no use if you have a hemorrhagic bleeding stroke. It would be a very bad idea to give an anticlotting drug if you are having a bleeding stroke.

The time window for identifying whether it is a good idea to give alteplase is about three hours. There is some evidence that longer than three hours is possible, but generally emergency rooms will not give the treatment after three hours. If you want to get in that three-hour window, a general piece of advice would be to look for a local hospital that has a PET scanner. For example, teaching hospitals at universities and at medical centers are usually better at this kind of thing than community hospitals. So some hospitals are able to diagnose and give an appropriate drug; others are not.

I have not mentioned other degenerative disorders in this lecture, but in a previous lecture I have mentioned Parkinson's disease, a loss of dopaminergic neurons. So there are other things that can also happen as we get older, relating to loss of neurons and loss of neural function.

Let's summarize what we have learned so far in this lecture. I have talked about adulthood and I have also talked about old age. The general principles are as follows. The first principle is that the brain changes throughout life, just as it does in childhood, adolescence, young adulthood, the brain continues to change as we get older. This change can take multiple forms. One form is change in synaptic strength as we have talked about in a previous lecture, but it can also take the form of the birth of new neurons, in some cases the loss of neurons, and also change in dendritic structure. So dendrites can change, for instance, they can branch, but also retract. These are changes that happen throughout life.

Another event that happens with age is functional change. So at the level of our behavior we can observe in ourselves and in others functional losses and some gains. So age is a mixed bag in which some things decline, other things perhaps increase a bit.

With some exceptions such as Alzheimer's disease, these losses and gains are a part of normal aging. Some of these changes happen quite early in life. So for instance, in the case of memory, peak function occurs fairly early around the age of 30, which accounts for why relatively early in life, in adulthood, people start reporting changes in memory function.

This gets us back to normal aging. Some of these losses experienced in aging are annoying, certainly annoying to me, as I get older; I am in my 40s. I will put it to you like this. When we are younger we can remember a lot of information. We can remember everybody's phone number. We can remember everybody's email address. We have a lot of capacity for memory.

Later these mental functions start to decline, as I have said. There are even everyday problems such as word-finding difficulty. There is a technical name, "anomic aphasia," which is also called "the Library of Congress effect." The memory will be retrieved eventually. It is just going to take forever.

So these kinds of problems are often annoying, and so people turn to ways of trying to stem or even reverse those changes. What I am going to do in the next lecture is I am going to talk about ways in which we attempt to preserve normal functioning and the efficacy of those strategies that we encounter.

"Brain Exercise" and Real Exercise
Lecture 23

> This activity that leads to larger changes is physical exercise, in other words, real exercise. ... Cicero, around 65 B.C., said, "It is exercise alone that supports the spirits and keeps the mind in vigor." ... [In contrast, it was] Mark Twain who said, "I take my only exercise acting as pallbearer at the funerals of my friends who exercise regularly." Clearly opinion is mixed from old times.

The aphorisms "use it or lose it," "sound mind and sound body," and "what's good for the heart is good for the brain" embody scientific findings that exercise, both mental and physical, really does help us retain cognitive functions as we age. We don't completely understand how this is so, but it's encouraging to know that we can take an active role in maintaining brain health for as long as possible.

Brain training, or mental exercise, is a hot topic and big business. By 2007, the brain training market was $80 million and growing. Puzzles, pattern recognition exercises, Sudoku and the like, along with working memory tasks, are purported to improve memory and other cognitive tasks—a claim neither strongly supported nor strongly refuted by scientific evidence. Practicing a brain exercise may improve your functioning in that particular task for a short while, but the benefit doesn't extend to other cognitive abilities. Improving your ability to remember a list of words, for example, does not improve spatial reasoning.

Some brain training is effective: It is often possible to get a more significant change in reaction time through brain training. One possibility is that reaction time is something that changes through natural biological mechanisms; it can also be trained through such exercises as playing video games.

Education helps retain cognitive abilities, possibly because it provides mental tools for engagement, helping us appreciate complexity in the world, enjoy art, or solve problems. Education gives us tools for thinking. An intellectually engaged lifestyle correlates with retained function in later life. Brain health benefits if you have multiple and complex hobbies (such as playing bridge), if you travel, learn a new language late in life, or learn musical instrument. An intellectually engaged lifestyle could help with our cognitive reserves, rather like gathering nuts for the winter.

Even more effective than brain-training exercises is physical exercise, particularly regular exercise maintained over a long period. Aerobic exercise is especially protective of brain functions. Exercise can ease depression, improve executive function (memory and planning), and dramatically reduce the risk of dementia—even when an exercise program isn't begun until middle age or much later. People with a sedentary lifestyle who adopt a regular exercise regimen in their 60s cut their risk of developing Alzheimer's by half.

> **Even more effective than brain-training exercises is physical exercise, particularly regular exercise maintained over a long period.**

Exercise does many things that could improve our cognitive abilities. It increases blood flow to the brain; triggers secretion of neurotrophic and atrophic factors, which improve dendritic growth; secretes naturally occurring opiates (endorphins); reduces stress hormone secretion; and improves cardiovascular health, which in turn reduces risk of stroke. The benefits of physical exercise last only up to a few weeks after the exercise ceases, however. You have to keep doing it, but you will see a large benefit. Other interventions that are good for the heart are also good for brain health. These include drinking red wine (in moderation), taking prescribed anti-clotting drugs, and eating brightly colored foods rich with antioxidants. ∎

Questions to Consider

1. What is the relative size of the benefit from brain training software compared with physical exercise? If you had $200 to spend on training software or on athletic gear/club membership, which would you choose?

2. What are the ways in which physical exercise might affect the brain?

"Brain Exercise" and Real Exercise
Lecture 23—Transcript

Welcome back. In the last lecture we talked about changes in the brain and changes in our mental capacities that come with age. Now what I would like to do in this lecture is talk about ways we can influence those changes, ways in which we can perhaps slow the effects of cognitive decline that happen as we get older. In particular, what we will do today in this lecture is talk about so-called "brain exercises." This is an increasingly popular product and we will talk about, in a critical way, ways in which and the extent of which brain exercises are genuinely useful. We will cover other things that have a potentially larger effect, including, surprisingly perhaps, real exercise.

Let's talk about what we are going to be doing today. We are going to be talking about cognitive changes associated with aging, mood, and other life events. We have covered that to a certain extent. What I am going to talk about is the popularity of brain training exercises and the peer-reviewed evidence of benefits in the scientific literature. I am going to compare that with the evidence in, again, peer-reviewed literature of benefits of physical exercise for brain function.

I am going to use a central measure that is very important to keep in mind when reading about these things in the paper, there is a central measure called "effect size" which is often neglected in popular accounts of these treatments. It is really important to think about effect size because it is a reflection of how likely you are to benefit. Finally I am going to talk about biological mechanisms by which these various manipulations that we try out can affect our brain function, so the biological mechanisms underlying all of these changes.

First off, let's think about the following question. What factors in surveys correlate with maintained mental function late in life? If we look in surveys of which factors seem to be associated with maintained mental function, the number one factor is education. The more education you have, the more you are able to retain cognitive function and mental abilities as you get older. That is an interesting phenomenon.

Higher education seems to be correlated with retained mental function. Why is that? There are two possible general explanations. One explanation is that higher education might give us mental tools for engagement. It might give us an ability to, say, appreciate complexity in the world, or to enjoy art, or to solve puzzles, or to engage in complex tasks. One possibility is that higher education gives us tools for thinking. Another possibility is that higher education is the province of people who are curious. It may be that curious people tend to stay in school longer. This is a chicken and egg problem.

The general observation seems to be that there is something about an intellectually engaged lifestyle which is correlated with retained function late in life. That extends not only to education but also to other mental activities. For example, other activities that may help you retain cognitive function are having multiple hobbies, having a complex hobby, say like playing bridge, traveling, learning a new language late in life, even though it is hard to learn a new language late in life, that would be an example of a mental activity that is challenging that can help you use your brain. There is a general sense from survey evidence that you should either use it or lose it. There is this idea that you should use your brain as you get older, and that seems to be correlated with retained function.

Another kind of activity that would be likely to help would be, for instance, learning to play a musical instrument. Now we are getting into a general principle that is reminiscent of what we heard about from childhood, the idea of active engagement. Something we encountered when we were talking about childhood seems to be the case also as we get older. Active engagement, active learning, seems to be important in retained mental function.

Another reason that intellectual engagement may help is something I mentioned before in the last lecture, the idea of a cognitive reserve. The general idea is that when you are learning about life and when you are doing things, you are gathering in some metaphorical sense, you are gathering nuts for winter. You are basically leading an intellectually engaged lifestyle and that builds up your cognitive capacities. Those capacities then serve you well as you get older and perhaps decline a little bit.

People have often tried to augment this by using exercises such as brain training. Brain training is a large market. As of 2007, a few years ago, the market for brain training software was about $80 million and it was growing. Brain training software consists of things that you can play on your home computer, you can play it on your Nintendo, or on you regular desktop computer, or even on a handheld device. These are pieces of software that go by names such as "Brain Age" or "Lumosity," pieces of software that help you maintain brain function or even augment brain function. They are basically puzzles you can do such as pattern recognition, that kind of thing, to help you keep your brain young. At least that is what the advertisements tell you.

Another example is Sudoku which typically costs very little, costs nothing. Sudoku puzzles are pattern completion puzzles where you have a grid of spaces. Those grids of spaces are divided into 3 x 3 sub-grids. What you do is you look for patterns and you look for completing patterns that fit in a square and perhaps are consistent with what you see in another square. These are pattern completion puzzles in which you sit there and try to work out what the hidden pattern is. That is an example of a puzzle that people do, again, in an attempt to keep their brains young.

I should say that I have nothing bad to say about Sudoku. I enjoy doing Sudoku puzzles and I have many friends who do. The question that I really want to get at now is the question of whether these products, such as these brain training products or Sudoku, whether they do any good. Advertising for these products often emphasizes the claim that they are designed by scientists or based on scientific research. The general idea is that there are laboratory studies that demonstrate that these products will keep your brain young. Perhaps a few may live up to this characterization. Certainly this is an area of active research.

I would say that many such claims are better characterized by what comedian Stephen Colbert calls "truthiness." What I mean by that is that they sound like truthful statements but if you look carefully, there is not very much evidence. What I would say, to be charitable, is that these are examples of exercises that are inspired by science but not necessarily proven by science. The reason is as follows. If you look very carefully at the literature results of whether these brain exercises do any good, there tend to be limitations. The limitations are that brain exercises, whatever they are, brain training, the benefits tend to be specific to the task practiced.

Let's think about what some of these exercises are like. Some of these tasks involve perhaps practicing your reaction time or perhaps looking at a list of things and trying to remember that list and that list of things would then build up your working memory. Perhaps it would be a puzzle in which you engage in spatial reasoning where you rotate an object mentally or where you try to determine the relationship of two things relative to one another in space. These are examples of tasks that are practiced by these pieces of software. They tend to train those skills.

What happens in these studies of these brain-training exercises is that when one practices these tasks, one tends to get better, but one tends to get better at that specific task. For instance, if you practice working memory, then you get better at working memory tasks but, say, you do not get better at a spatial reasoning task. Likewise if you get better at Sudoku, you are not going to get better at your working memory. The fact that these benefits tend to be specific to the task means that unless your activities that you are practicing span a broad spectrum of abilities, then there is not necessarily a proven general benefit to these mental fitness programs.

The idea that any single brain exercise program late in life can act as a quick fix for general mental function is almost entirely faith based. I should say, as a caveat, that it is admittedly hard to design studies to prove that brain gyms work, these pieces of brain training. One big problem is that they typically require many hours of training. You have to practice these things for hours over several weeks. What that does is that it gives people a strong desire to believe that they have not wasted their money or wasted their time. That motivation can cause a placebo-like affect in which after training, participants may put more effort or attention into doing well in the tests than they did before training. There is some problem with a lot of these studies because you have to control for such placebo effects.

To control for placebo effects, a comparison group must be given an ineffective form of training that requires an equivalent amount of work. The idea in an effective test of brain training is that you have to have a test group and a control group. That is a condition that is rarely, if ever, met. A lot of the published evidence is not really all that good for, or for that matter, against brain training.

Let's consider a specific example. Let's ask the question: Can brain training ever make you smarter, actually increase your IQ? This is not really demonstrated. Here is why. Intelligence tests attempt to measure something called "fluid intelligence," the ability to solve problems. Problem solving typically involves holding information in memory and then manipulating the information. For instance, a logic puzzle where, say, Albert is sitting to the right of the dentist. The dentist is not Mrs. Brown. Mrs. Brown is across from the turkey, or whatever it might be. These logic puzzles are puzzles in which we have to manipulate information and solve some complex puzzle.

It has been observed that working memory correlates with fluid intelligence. It has also been observed that you can build up working memory through practice. If you can build up working memory through practice, and working memory correlates with fluid intelligence, so could it be that working memory practice can build up problem solving intelligence? It turns out that the evidence is not in yet. It turns out that there are problems with some of the experiments that have been done to date. The problems involve things like a test practice effect or some kind of placebo effect that I just described. It may well be that, in fact, it is possible to increase intelligence through some kind of practice, but it has not really been very well demonstrated.

Now what I want to do is address a key question which is the question of, how large are the benefits of these exercises? So far I have told you about how the exercise benefits tend to be specific to a particular task and not generalized to other tasks. One important question you should always ask when reading about some treatment is, how large is the effect? How likely would you be to get a benefit in your everyday life? Would you notice?

I should say that this is very different from the criterion of, say, publishability in a scientific journal. If you look in a group and you look in another group, it is certainly possible that you can see a statistically-significant difference between the two groups. But how large is the effect because, of course, each group can have a distribution, you can have a range of performance in one group and a range of performance in another group or the same group after testing after practice.

The question is, how large is the size of the effect? That tells you whether and by how much you would plausibly expect a benefit. This question of how large the size of the effect is is usually overlooked in news stories probably because it requires a small amount of statistical knowledge. Unfortunately it is unlikely that you are going to encounter effect sizes very much in the news articles that you read or that you hear about on the radio or watch on television or read about online. But at least I want to give you the idea of an effect size so you can get a sense of whether something is likely to be larger or smaller, at least the things I am talking about today. Then if you are really industrious, you can go look up effect sizes in the library.

The key concept that you need to understand in order to understand the concept of effect size is the concept of the standard deviation. The standard deviation is a statistical measure of the amount of variation in a group. For instance, on the famous bell-shaped curve, we all know that many distributions fall in a bell-shaped curve. It turns out that about 2/3 of the data points in a bell-shaped curve are within one standard deviation above or below the average. Bell-shaped curves intrinsically have a shape in which about two-thirds of people, say, who take a test are within one standard deviation of the average.

The effect size is defined as in units of standard deviation, how far you are from the control group. For instance, if you have an experimental group and a control group—one group that did a brain exercises and one group that did not, or one group after brain exercise and one group before—if you take the difference between those two groups and you ask what is the difference in average between the two groups, and then you divide that by the standard deviation, that is the effect size. For instance, if there is no effect at all, then the effect size is 0. If there is a change, then the effect gets larger and larger and can be 1 or 2 or whatever.

This effect size, which is in units of standard deviation, can be interpreted as follows. Roughly speaking, think of effect size as being, say, 0.2, 0.5, and 0.8.

An effect size of 0.2 is what is referred to as a small effect size. For instance, to relate it to everyday life, an effect size of 0.2 corresponds to the difference between the heights of 15-year-old girls in the U.S and 16-year-old girls in the US. That is a small effect and, in fact, you would have difficulty telling a girl's age just from her height. A medium effect size of 0.5 corresponds to the difference between the heights of, say, 14-year-old girls and 18-year-old girls. Finally, a large effect size, one of 0.8, equates to the difference between the heights of 13-year-old girls and 18-year-old girls. That is just a way of getting a feeling for what a small, medium, or large effect size is.

Let's consider one of the papers that claims a benefit from brain training software. This is a typical paper. A typical benefit from brain training software, after weeks of practice, is an effect size of 0.25. Now, 0.25 is in the category of small. I gave it to you in units of, say, teenage girls. Another example would be if you are in a group of 20. Let's say that you're average in a group of 20, you would be at around number 10 or 11. An effect size of 0.25 takes you from number 10 in the group to about number 8 in the group. That is obviously not exactly an impressive effect. That is the effect size of the training of the task to its own task. That is, therefore, the largest effect you are going to see when doing some kind of brain training. It turns out that cross training effects are nearly nonexistent. In fact, that improvement from number 10 to number 8 is, in fact, hardly any at all.

A larger effect, the medium and large effects that I mentioned, are going from number 10 to number 6 or even to number 4. Now we are getting into territory where it is a pretty good change because if we could get a change that took us from number 10 out of a group of 20 to number 4, we would take it. This is not true of all brain training. There are exceptions to this rule.

There is one particular exception which is reaction time. It is often possible to get a more significant change in reaction time through brain training. That is interesting, for instance, as people get older, their reaction time slows, so it is possible, for example, to get a significant improvement in reaction time. One marketed audience for people who take these brain training exercises is driving safety. For instance, if you can get your reaction time down, then perhaps your stopping distance would be shorter and you would be a somewhat safer driver.

Reaction time slows in the old probably having to do with things like the speed in neuro-processing, in particular for instance, the speed of long distance conduction of signals. Remember that there is an insulating sheath on axons, it is called "myelin." Myelin replacement continues throughout life but, in fact, slows down in the 40s. One possibility is that reaction time is something that changes through natural biological mechanisms and can also be retrained by video games such as brain training for reaction time.

We have talked about brain training and these pieces of software that you can buy or perhaps get for free. Now what I want to do is to contrast that with another activity, an activity that leads to larger changes. This activity that leads to larger changes is physical exercise, in other words, real exercise. These are ideas that have been around for a while. They have been quoted by ancients who were not scientists. I will give you a few examples. Cicero around 65 B.C. said, "It is exercise alone that supports the spirits and keeps the mind in vigor." Another example comes from the second president of the United States, John Adams, who said, "Exercise invigorates and enlivens all the faculties of body and of mind. It spreads a gladness and a satisfaction over our minds, and qualifies us for every sort of business and every sort of pleasure." Opinions from previous times are not unanimous. I will give you a third one which is Mark Twain who said, "I take my only exercise acting as pallbearer at the funerals of my friends who exercise regularly." Opinion was mixed in previous times.

Let's look at the peer-reviewed evidence. What is interesting about the peer-reviewed evidence is that the effects of physical activity are, in fact, rather large. The effect size is what I previously called "a medium sized effect size." If you look at work, for instance, in reviewed literature from Kolken and Kramer the effect size is 0.5 to 0.6 standard deviations. This is a medium size effect. It is an effect that you might very well notice in your everyday life. In some cases, the effect is even larger.

Here is the summary of what has been found. Exercise, especially aerobic exercise of the type that gets your heart rate up, is strongly protective of brain functions. The effect is largest if you are active starting in middle age. If you start exercising in middle age, that is great. However, even if you start exercise later in life, in your 70s, that still improves the executive function.

Recall, I have talked about executive function before. The things that have been measured that are improved are working memory, making plans, acting on those plans. The effective amount of exercise in reaping these benefits is about 30 minutes at a time, enough to get your heart rate up, several times a week. That is enough exercise to protect your brain.

It turns out that exercise of this type, whether started in middle age or in late life, reduces the risk of dementia. People who exercise regularly starting from middle age are 1/3 as likely to get Alzheimer's disease in their 70s. If they start in their 60s, the risk drops by half. Exercise changes not only the risk of normal aging, but also reduces the risk of dementia. It is good for both normal and pathological function.

This great benefit, how does it work? Well, it turns out that exactly how exercise works on the brain is not fully worked out. There are possibilities for how it can help. One possibility is that exercise, just as it improves cardiovascular function, can lead to increased blood flow, can improve the flow of blood into the brain. Another possibility is that exercise can trigger the secretion of what are called "neurotrophic factors." These are secreted factors in the brain that can lead to growth, atrophic factor, growth, triggering factor, is something that can cause, for instance, dendritic growth, dendritic sprouting.

In addition to increased blow flow, exercise may increase the secretion of neurotrophic factors, one of them is called "brain-derived neurotrophic factor," in other words "BDNF." Another possibility is that there can be other biochemical changes that happen in the brain. For instance, it has been demonstrated that exercise causes the secretion of naturally-occurring opiates, endorphins, endocannabinoids are also secreted. Serotonin levels change. Finally, exercise can reduce stress. There are different things that exercise can do that can alter brain signaling ranging from opiate secretion to decreased stress hormone secretion.

All of these converge on a couple of common cellular targets. One of them is the survival of neurons, and even in some cases the growth of dendrites. So that is on possible outcome of exercise. Another possibility is the reduced risk of stroke that comes from having a healthier cardiovascular system. These kinds of mechanisms are ways in which exercise may act upon the brain.

Now I want to talk about ways in which physical exercise may differ from brain training. The downside of an exercise program is that the observed benefits of exercise typically last about as long as the exercise program or perhaps some weeks afterwards. That is opposed to brain training whose effects are long lasting. What that suggests is that there is a difference in the mechanism of brain training benefits and exercise benefits. Mainly it goes as follows.

Brain training is likely to rely on plasticity mechanisms. I have talked repeatedly about this principle of activity affecting synaptic strength, affecting brain capacity, this Hebb principle. The positive effect of brain training is that it is likely to draw upon those mechanisms, and the effects of brain training can last for years. That is likely because they rely on changes in brain circuitry. In other words, changes in brain connections which include various forms of change in synapses and neurons that are use-dependent can last you a long time. Even though the effects of brain training are small and even though they are perhaps hard to notice in everyday life, they do have the advantage of lasting.

The same would be true for another capacity that we talked about some lectures ago, another capacity that can be built up with practice, namely willpower. So there are certain kinds of training, because they rely on the use of a neural circuit, that would be likely to last even if the effects are not so large.

Now contrast that with an exercise program. We have been talking about physical exercise. Physical exercise may confer benefits that depend on things such as blood flow. These are benefits that do not far out last the time that you stop exercising. They last as long as the improvements to your cardiovascular system persist. The problem with exercise is that you have to keep on doing it. So that is a downside of exercise but you will experience a large benefit.

Let's talk about some other benefits of exercise for the brain. There have been some changes in the recommendations from the United States Department of Health and Human Services. These recommendations center around the frequency and intensity of exercise that is likely to improve brain function although they do not couch it that way. Health and Human Services has suggested that adults aged 18 to 64 should do 2 ½ hours a week of moderate intensity or 1 hour 15 minutes, 75 minutes, a week of vigorous intensity aerobic physical activity, or some equivalent combination of moderate and vigorous aerobic physical activity. They say that these episodes of aerobic activity should be performed in episodes of at least 10 minutes, preferably spread throughout the week. They are fairly specific about this and this is a significant increase from previous recommendations from the United States federal government.

It turns out that they also list in their brochure, which I encourage you to go read on their website, they describe the benefits that come from physical exercise for the old and also for the young. What I want to do is I just want to talk about specifically the benefits for brain function. The specific benefits include improvements, as I said to cardiovascular function, but also reduction of depression. For instance, the symptoms of depression can be reduced by exercise. Also they point out that there is improved cognitive function as I have pointed out to you.

What they have also pointed out is that these benefits of exercise extend not only to the old but also to younger people. So children and adolescents also have better cardiovascular function, better bone health, better body composition. Interestingly, there is some evidence that exercise can even influence anxiety and depression in the young. Exercise can reduce symptoms of anxiety and depression in young people. That is very interesting. What it suggests is that physical exercise is good at all ages.

Let's back up a little bit. I have told you that exercise's effects are larger than the effects of brain training. I have told you that exercise's effects are also effective on multiple brain functions. There is an interesting question that comes up here. Is there a general principle that can help us identify other interventions that are good for brain function? The answer to that question is yes.

The answer is that there is a general principle which is that interventions that are good for the heart are also found to be good for the brain as well. I will give you a few examples. One example is certain kinds of alcoholic beverage. It turns out that alcohol is not damaging to the brain in moderate amounts. For instance, there is an old joke that alcohol kills brain cells, that turns out not to be true. There is a safe amount of alcohol. That safe amount of alcohol is up to about two alcoholic drinks a day in men, about one drink a day in women, some studies say that it might be somewhat higher.

Not only is it true that alcohol does not kill brain cells, but it turns out that certain forms of alcoholic beverages can, in fact, be neuro-protective. That is, in particular, red wines, not liquor, not white wine, not beer. Specifically the beverage that has some neuro-protective effect is red wine. It turns out that study was done, one influential study was done, at the University of Bordeaux in France. It turns out that result has replicated by other studies done in non-wine producing regions.

How is it that red wine protects the brain? It turns out that the mechanism is not fully understood. There is one compound that has been identified in red wine in grape skins called "resveratrol." Resveratrol has been shown to have some protective benefit. It is probably not the case that resveratrol is the only thing in red wine that helps because the equivalent amount, if you give it to rats, you can get a certain amount of benefit in the rats, but the amount of resveratrol that the rats have to consume is equivalent to about 3,000 bottles of wine per day. That is clearly more than the typical serving and more than the two drinks a day that I mentioned before, a lot more.

What that suggests is that there must be other compounds in red wine that confer some kind of neuro-protective benefit. There is evidence that some of these benefits can come from drinking not just wine, but also grape juice. That is not as much fun but it shows that there is something in red wine, probably in grape skins, that confer some kind of benefit for brain function.

Another example of the good-for-the-heart-good-for-the-brain principle is anti-clotting drugs. Drugs such as aspirin and ibuprofen, these are drugs that are demonstrated to reduce the decline in cognitive function and also reduce the incidence of dementia and stroke. These blood-thinning drugs, these anti-clotting drugs, seem to have some kind of neuro-protective effect.

Finally we have antioxidant foods. These include things that are rich in antioxidants; they include other brightly colored foods. I will give you examples of antioxidant foods: blueberries, omega-3 fatty acid such as found in say salmon, and brightly colored foods such as you would find in leafy vegetable or in carrots. All of these foods demonstrated effects on cardiovascular health. These types of foods have also been demonstrated to have protective effects on cognitive ability. So these are all ways in which things that you can do that are good for your heart are also good for your brain.

Let's know look at what we have learned today. Let's summarize. Firstly, I have told you that brain training exercises may have long-lasting effects but those effects are small. They are limited to the task practiced. As of today, the scientific evidence for their benefits is not yet fully strong; it is not yet strong evidence. I have also told you that a stronger intervention is physical exercise. Physical exercise has been demonstrated to influence executive function. It is not known what the mechanism is, but the mechanism might be increases in blood flow to the brain and perhaps the secretion of neurotrophic factors and other neurochemicals.

There is a general principle which is that things that are good for your heart and cardiovascular system are also good for your brain. In general, if we think about this, there is a general principle that applies here which is that intellectual engagement and physical activity are major principles for retaining function as well as heart health. In short, a sound mind in a sound body. That is obviously very old wisdom, but it turns out that there is current medical evidence for that.

I want to congratulate all of you who are covering all of your bases. Ideally you will be watching this lecture while you are on the treadmill. If you are doing that, then you are covering both ends of things. So get on the treadmill. In the next lecture what we will do is we will turn to animal and human personality.

Animal and Human Personality
Lecture 24

It is possible to take personality tests of these same types that are applied to animals and give them to people, as well. In fact, of course, they are more prevalent in human psychology because it turns out that there is much more of an interest in human personality than there is in octopus personality.

The brain factor that differentiates us from one another is personality, a strongly inheritable property that is determined by hundreds of gene combinations and by environmental influences—but hardly at all, it turns out, by parents.

Personality, or temperament, is a difficult thing to study because it's not quantifiable; that is, it can't be measured or scored. Still, we have a powerful tendency to impute motivation to other people and even to other things. Scientists have studied animal behavior and catalogued individual traits in an attempt to understand the biological reasons for them. These ethologists discovered that certain traits tend to go together in clusters. For example, the cluster traits for extroversion include sociability, outgoingness, and assertiveness. Two important personality tests are used to assess specific traits. The five-factor model (FFM) assesses openness to experience, conscientiousness, extroversion, agreeableness, and neuroticism, all of which show strong inheritability. The Meyers-Briggs test classifies traits into four categories.

What is the reason for so much variation in personality? Individual traits can be an advantage or a disadvantage depending on environmental conditions. Great variation gives the population in general a greater chance of survival no matter the environmental conditions. For example, a daring animal would get more food and be more successful with a low density of predators, but that same daring trait would increase the animal's chance of falling prey if there was a higher density of predators. In that situation, the more timid animals that are content to eat scraps and avoid predators would have a better survival rate.

There seems to be a 30% to 50% inheritable component to personality and a 50% to 70% environmental component. We don't know what causes environment-induced personality development, and we haven't identified specific genes that cause specific personality traits. Instead, clusters of genes, perhaps hundreds of clusters, make up an individual trait, making them polygenic.

Anxiety is associated with shortage of a specific protein responsible for the uptake of serotonin, a neuromodulator involved in mood.

Half the variation of anxiety is inherited. Anxiety is associated with shortage of a specific protein responsible for the uptake of serotonin, a neuromodulator involved in mood. But this protein plays a small role. Novelty-seeking involves dopamine receptors. Dopamine and serotonin activity seem to have some role in predicting personality, but the contribution they make so far seems to be small. These findings point to the possibility of understanding how personality is determined by genes and by the environment. The mechanisms of personality are still a mystery, and the focus is on neurotransmitters. This topic is only just beginning to unfold.

Personality starts to manifest itself when a baby is about 3 months old; from there, a combination of innate mechanisms and individual experience influences the eventual outcome of personality development. Parents really have little influence over their children's personalities, except when a child is shy or anxious. Shy babies may be shy toddlers and children, but this tendency usually diminishes. A very small minority persist in this behavior into adulthood, where they have a high risk of anxiety disorders. However, parents who are calm and nurturing can help teach the shy or anxious child important coping skills to overcome these difficulties and become successful adults.

Personality changes as we grow, staying malleable until about the age of 30, when it becomes more stable. It is most stable between the ages of 50 to 70. ■

1. How much can parents influence a child's personality development after he or she is born?

2. In what cases can a parent have an important positive influence on a child's temperament?

Animal and Human Personality

Lecture 24—Transcript

Welcome back. We have talked so far about developmental stages and life stages that we all share. Now what I want to do is I want to start talking about the topic of individuality. In particular, I want to start talking about the brain factors, the features of our brains that make us different from one another. What I would like to talk about today is one of those things, a major thing that distinguishes us from each other and that is personality.

What I would like to do is cover the topic of personality, the biology and the phenomenological aspects of personality. I would like to start from a place that is a good place to begin when we want to talk about something that perhaps is a little bit hard to get a handle on, I want to start with animals. What I would like to do today is start talking about temperament in animals' personality, talk about the genetics of personality, and in particular the neural mechanisms that may underlie personality and what we know about the neural mechanisms, and environmental influences in personality. Finally, I would like to end with some practical information for parents and perhaps for offspring as well.

First let's get a sense for whether personality, this thing that perhaps may seem a little bit soft, to get a handle on whether personality can be studied in a scientific manner. One way to ask that question is to see how it is investigated in animals where perhaps we are a little bit separated from our own interests in the subject. It turns out that the study of personality in animals has come up more and more in the last few years. That was not the case, say, in the decades previously. Many traditional psychologists previously had avoided the study of studying the differences among animals altogether. It was thought that perhaps what we should be doing is studying how animals are all the same. For instance consider the pioneer in animal behavioral research, B.F. Skinner. B.F. Skinner made a point of giving tests to animals under conditions that made the responses as reliable as possible. His experiments were designed to keep conditions always the same, the famous Skinner box. The Skinner box was designed to remove any distracting stimuli that might lead to environmental variation.

In this Skinner box a perfect experiment would be one in which there is no variation from an individual to an individual so whatever animal you put into the box, you would get the same result no matter what. In principle, what that meant was a really good experiment with one animal was enough to reach conclusion, and that perhaps you would do a second animal just to make sure that everything was OK and that there were no technical problems. The general idea here was to study behavior in a way that individuality was not part of the experiment.

One major thread running through behavioral approaches to psychology at that time, and even now, is that one should limit investigations to directly observable behaviors. The problem with personality was thought to be that if you cannot directly observe it then it is subjective and you cannot score it, and therefore it is not possible to objectively study personality. There is truth to this. For instance, we are constantly mapping our own actions to our individual motives, our own preferences, and we tend to assign similar motives and preferences to the actions of others. There is that powerful tendency for us to impute motivation to other people and even to other things. This is a general framework called "theory of mind." We are going to be talking about theory of mind again in a later lecture, when we start talking about the social brain.

For example, it is common to talk about not only living things but also non-living things as having personalities. For instance, it is common to describe a car as being temperamental or perhaps a house as being personal and inviting. Yet it is quite clear, in these cases, that nobody would ever attribute literal personality to these objects because they are not alive. That was the objection.

A different approach has come up in the last few years. It comes from a field called "ethology." Ethology is the scientific study of animal behavior. Ethologists tend to emphasize natural situations and they are also very interested in differences among individual animals. Like behaviorists, ethologists are interested in direct observations, they are interested in behaviors, but they are specifically interested in individual observations of one animal in context and then watching another animal. So they will ask things like, in a spontaneous or natural situation, they will ask questions like, did the animal attack, did it retreat, did it curl up in a corner? Ethologists' interests in natural differences have enabled them to catalog individual traits in a rigorous way and to try to understand the biological reasons for them. It is really in this discipline that the study of animal personality has really developed and blossomed in the last few years.

Now we can ask the question, if you are an ethologist, how would you study personality in animals? Sometimes the word "personality" is used, other times the word "temperament" is used, but the general question is the same. How do you study individual differences in reactions of animals to a situation? There are two major approaches that an ethologist can take. One approach is to ask the keeper of the animals. Just ask people who spend a lot of time in the company of those animals, what did the animal do. Another way to do it is to observe the animals directly and to make observations, as I mentioned before, did the animal attack and so on.

Let's consider asking the keepers. If you ask the keeper to score animals, what you can do is you can ask people who are familiar with an animal to say will you please look for essential traits, such as fearfulness, aggressiveness, affability or calmness, traits that can exist outside of cognition yet are clearly and repeatedly apparent in different individual animals in varying measures. The idea is that if you look at individuals within a species, you might see more affability or less affability in an individual and it is something that varies within the species.

One classic study was done on hyenas. This is a study done on dozens of hyenas. Four caretakers of this hyena colony were asked to, independently without looking at each other's answers, to independently fill out questionnaires about each individual hyena. What they were given was a modified version of a widely applied human personality test. These caretakers were given a questionnaire saying well, what do you know about that hyena over there? The caretakers' assessments often agreed with one another. They often converged, as is the case for assessments done on human personality. Individual caretakers would come up with the same rating of an individual hyena in regard to excitability or sociability, curiosity, assertiveness. These are traits that you can also see in our own species. These caretakers scored individual hyenas in the same way.

That is one way that it is possible to determine that individual animals can vary from one another. The other way, as I mentioned, is to observe the animals directly. It is possible to do this. In particular, there is a classic study that is a landmark in the study of animal personality done by Anderson and Mather. This is a paper that came out in 1993. What they did is they studied the Great Pacific octopuses. They looked at these octopuses and looked at their reactions to situations presented to the octopuses. In particular, they found that individual octopus reactions could be categorized into three major dimensions. One dimension is reactivity, another dimension is activity, and the third dimension is avoidance. What they found was that these three dimensions, each of which could vary more or less, were sufficient to describe tendencies of individual octopuses. What they did is they did experiments like they would have a human observer stick her face into the tank and see what the octopus did, or they would take a test tube cleaning brush, a small cleaning brush, and put it near the animal and see whether the animal retreated or attacked it or they would throw a tasty crab into the water and see whether the octopus went for it. What they observed was individual octopuses had predictable responses. Some octopuses were very bold and went for the crab, others did not.

It turns out that these kinds of tests, now, are applicable both to animals and to humans. It is possible to take personality tests of these same types that are applied to animals and give them to people as well. In fact, of course, they are more prevalent in human psychology because it turns out that there is much more of an interest in human personality than there is in octopus personality, which I guess depends on what you like.

The most widely applied personality test in humans is something called "the Five-Factor Model," the "F.F.M." It is a very popular model for describing personality. The typical personality test will look for these five factors. The five factors are openness to experience, conscientiousness, extroversion, agreeableness, and neuroticism. Those are the five factors that are typically tested for. Each of these dimensions includes recognizable traits that tend to go together. When you give a test to people, there are certain traits that tend to go together. These are called by statisticians' "clusters" and also I have used the word "dimensions." So there are certain traits that seem to go together and those are often called "clusters." For example, cluster traits for extroversion. For instance, an extroverted person would be more sociable, outgoing, and assertive. In the dimension of neuroticism, a neurotic person would be more anxious, moody, and stressed. Those things tend to go with one another.

Another popular test that is often given, this is one that you can find online on the internet, is the Myers-Briggs test. This is a very popular personality test that one can take to find out whether you are EMTJ or whatever. So there are these four categories that you can score on the Myers-Briggs test. It is a way to find out about personality types.

That is how you measure personality, now let's step back a bit and start talking about the biology of personality. First let's talk about it just a little bit from an evolutionary point of view. One question that one can ask is, what is the point of an individual variation? What is the reason for variation to exist in a population? It turns out that these individual traits that we have talked about can be advantageous or disadvantageous depending on environmental conditions. I will give you an example. One example is extroversion. Extroverted people seem to have a selection advantage. In other words, they get more dates, they are more likely to find a mate, and they are more likely to reproduce. From a classic evolutionary standpoint, extroverted people have a selection advantage. It also turns out that extroverted people go out and do stuff. They have been shown in studies to have more accidents and also to be more likely to end up in the hospital. These are people who can get the mates as long as they can avoid having accidents along the way.

If we look at animals, we can see a similar property in animals. Daring animals get more food. They are more likely to get out there and grab the crab that is out there in the open. They also have a larger chance of themselves becoming food, of being eaten. You can imagine, then, in a situation where there is a low density of predators then these daring animals get more food. But if the predator density is high, then the advantage goes to the stay-at-homes who can hunt for scraps after the predators are gone and perhaps they will have a higher survival advantage. That is an example of which extroversion or rather, willingness to get out there and grab food, might be advantageous in one circumstance and not in another.

There is a particularly interesting example of this which is the North American fishing spider. This is a spider that has, again, individual variation. Some fishing spiders are extremely aggressive hunters. They are always the first to grab passing food. You would think that would be an advantage and there is an advantage food-wise. It turns out that there is a strong disadvantage in these spiders during mating season. What happens is that during mating season, they cannot keep their legs off their suitors but they eat them before they have a chance to mate. As a result there is a strong selection disadvantage because if you eat your partner then that is pretty much the end of the line.

There is another possible reason for individual personality to vary in a population. This is something that is a bit of a controversial concept in evolutionary biology. The general idea is that conditions vary from generation to generation. That is known to be the case, that is not controversial. If conditions vary from generation to generation then it is possible that a range of personalities in any given generation might optimize the likelihood that some member of that generation will make it to the next generation. The idea here would be that natural variation of the population is an advantageous trait at the whole species level. The reason this is controversial is that evolutionary biologists do not like to talk about some selection, some advantage, that happens at a group level. The concept of group selection is something that is thought to be unlikely in terms of inheritance. The exception to that is cases in which biological trait is carried by many genes. As opposed to one gene, such as eye color or something simple like that, personality seems to be determined by many genes. I will come to that in a moment. So that would be the way in which this group property could be passed on from generation to generation.

Now let's come to that question, genetics and also environmental contributors to personality. Let's ask the question, is personality an inheritable trait? Again, let's start from animals and then work to people. A good case in point is the case of dairy goats. This is a very nice study in which dairy goats were paired. There are pairs of dairy goat siblings separated at birth. In these pairs of siblings, one set of siblings was raised by goats, in a regular goat family, and then the other set of siblings was raised by humans. The idea was that the humans would interact with the goats, work with them every day, feed them, handle them every day. You have one group of goat siblings raised by goats and then their brothers and sisters raised by humans.

What was found was that in each of these groups, timidity was measured. Timidity was measured both by timidity with a human person, so for instance, if you stand in front of the goat, or for instance a non-human thing, like say for instance, exposing the goat to a yearling goat put in the pen or reaction to the gate being left open. What was found was that in each group, the rank order of timidity is the same. "Rank order" means that some goats were more timid than others. What was observed was that there was an order of timidity from most timid to least timid. The ordering was the same in siblings. If two goats were siblings raised by goats or humans, they tended to be about as timid as one another and more timid than the others in that group. However, there was a general tendency for human-raised goats to be less timid than their goat-raised counterparts. In general, the goat-raised goat would be more timid than the human-raised goat, but within each group the rank ordering was the same.

What this shows is something a little bit complicated. It shows that there is a role for genetics for inherited tendencies but also that there is a role for environment. In the case of genetics, the fact that the rank ordering is the same suggests that siblings share something in common with one another, yet rearing by human can lead to less timidity to a variety of situations including non-human stimulus. What that suggests is that there is a roll for genes in environment in setting personality, at least this one particular personality trait, in goats.

This turns out to be true for other traits as well and it also true, in particular, in us, in humans. Remember I talked about the Five-Factor Model. It turns out that all five factors in the personality inventory show strong inheritability. What that means is that people who are more closely related to one another are more likely to share personality traits. For instance, identical twins are more likely to share personality traits than non-identical twins and siblings and more distant relatives. What that means is that there is a genetic component in personality. And what that means, for instance, is that each one of you shares quite a few personality traits in common with your biological parents, that tends to be true, and that sharing a personality trait with your biological parents is true even if you are adopted, even if you have never met your parents, you will share some personality traits with that person. This is commonly reported anecdotally when people met their biological parents after many years.

The general observation is that all five personality axes are strongly heritable. This inheritability is 30 percent to 50 percent of the variation that is seen, and can be attributed to genetics. So that is almost as strong as the heritability, say, of intelligence. Personality is a fairly strongly inheritable property. I have talked about the environmental component with the goats. The fact that there are 30 percent to 50 percent heritable personality traits means that there is, in fact, 50 percent to 70 percent environmental component. That means that as we grow up, as we develop and grow up, there are contributions to our personality that vary somewhat independently or that can diverge from our initial genetic endowment. It turns out that this is a bit of a mystery.

What causes environmentally induced personality development is hard to identify. One obvious candidate is parenting. Parents love to think that they can influence their children's personalities but it turns out that it is probably not parenting because identical twins are about as similar as twins reared apart. If you separate twins and raise them in different families, there is still a lot of similarity between the personalities. It seems like there is some other environmental influence. It turns out that it is not known what that influence is. For example, it could be school; it could be the peer group. After all, those are people that kids look to for examples for how to behave. It could be simply chance events. What is interesting here is that parents have relatively little influence over how their children develop personality-wise. That is interesting and perhaps a good tip for people raising children that you are not going to have a whole lot of influence over your child's personality.

Now let's talk about the genetics of personality a little bit, get into the details. I have said that personality is inheritable but it turns out that inborn aspects of personality traits are polygenic. What that means is that they are constructed from the action of many genes, perhaps hundreds. There is not such a thing as an aggression gene or an affability gene. Rather, it is the interaction of many genes working together. What that means is that people have difficulty looking for the genetic causes of personality traits. For example, even in the best cases where it is well worked out, genetic traits, such as particular receptor types in the brain or specific transporters of neurotransmitters have so far only been able to account for a small fraction of the variation seen from an individual to an individual. What it means is that the genetic studies that have been done so far are, in fact, large enough to lead to the ability to get published in a nice scientific journal but not necessarily large enough to account for a lot of our everyday experience. It is good for the scientist but maybe less good for us trying to understand our everyday lives. I will give you a few examples.

Here is one example, the trait of anxiety. In identical twins, about half the variation in anxiety-related personality traits is inherited. For example, anxiety-related personality traits are associated with a shortage of a specific protein, this has been shown, that when one does human genetic linkage analysis that there is a shortage of a specific protein that is responsible for the reuptake of serotonin.

Serotonin is a neuro-modulator that is released that seems to be involved in mood. Serotonin reuptake is the target of Prozac. Remember that Prozac is a blocker of selective serotonin reuptake. It turns out that this protein seems to be linked somehow to anxiety. There is a linkage but it also turns out that the influence of this reuptake protein, when you look at the natural variation of the protein, accounts for less than a tenth of the inheritable variation in anxiety. What that means is then, in fact, very little of the variation of anxiety is explainable by this particular protein.

Just an aside on Prozac, one thing that is interesting is that it treats anxiety and depression and it does so by blocking the serotonin reuptake protein. That is in the wrong direction because I just said that low reuptake protein is associated with more anxiety. So how is it that Prozac could possibly work by blocking it? That is funny, what is probably going on here, what is likely, is partly explained by the fact that Prozac takes weeks to work. You have to take it for a long period of time before it has an effect. What that implies is that what Prozac is probably doing is that it is probably inducing plasticity. It is probably inducing change in the brain, specifically in the serotonin-signaling system. For example, Prozac might lead to lots of serotonin release or lots of serotonin hanging around after it is released. That perhaps would lead to some kind of adaptive response, for instance, desensitization of serotonin signaling pathways and then weaken the strength of those pathways. That would be an example in which this little bit of knowledge that we have about personality can be used and can account for something that happens in a common drug treatment. That is one example of a linkage between a molecule in signaling and in personality.

Here is another example for genetics and personality. There are some efforts that have been made in understanding novelty seeking. Novelty seeking is the tendency to seek out new experiences. What has been observed is that novelty seeking also has genetic linkage. It is possible to find genes that seem to be associated. In particular, there are variations in particular types of dopamine receptor genes that seem to co-vary in a way that can predict novelty seeking. Again, that is a linkage that is present in the population, if you look in enough people, but in fact the amount of variation explained is very small. It seems like a robust result because it has been observed in humans, and also as it turns out, in thoroughbred horses. Nonetheless, it is only a small amount of the total amount of variation.

To summarize, if we were to try to take a strongly genetic approach to personality, if we wanted to really understand individual genes, the beginnings of this field are that dopamine and serotonin activity seem to have some role in predicting personality. But it turns out that the contribution that they make is only small so far. What is exciting about these findings is not that dopamine receptors or serotonin reuptake are key determinates of personality, although they make an important contribution. The interesting thing about these findings is they point to the possibility of understanding how personality is determined by genes and also by the environment. That future possibility, I think, is quite exciting. So far what we have done is we, the field of neuroscience, have done is look at obvious molecules such as serotonin and dopamine-related molecules. That is an obvious starting point and it has gotten to a certain level of progress.

One difficulty of the neuroscience of personality then is that we do not actually know what the mechanisms are. The focus has been on neurotransmitters because pharmacology has been pretty successful at taking a hammer to personality. The idea that one can really alter one's presented personality with drugs like Prozac or even something like, say, cocaine. Those can alter affect, alter personality, but in fact there is a lot of other stuff going on inside the brain. There is stuff inside cells, say, intracellular signaling, inside cells where biochemical messengers are generated or perhaps at the network level. Drugs are not necessarily good at tweaking details at these levels either inside cells or, say, in the whole network. So there seems to be a lot more that needs to be learned there before we can really get a handle on the mechanisms of personality.

When people talk about the neurochemistry of personality, it is clear that we are at the beginning of this topic and that it is going to require better genetics, biochemistry perhaps, and understanding networks of signaling neurons.

Now I want to come back to the environmental topic, environmental influences on personality. I alluded to this by talking about parents. There is a common myth. The common myth is what I could call "the blank slate myth," the idea that parents can influence a child's personality. It turns out that parents find out, if they are paying attention, that they are wrong. Techniques that work so well for soothing one infant, inexplicably fail to calm the second one. Or you raise your child and you discover that no matter what you want your child to do, that little boy is going to start playing war with sticks or toy guns, or that little girl is going to get interested in dolls or pink frilly dresses. It turns out that there are innate tendencies that are very hard to influence from a parenting standpoint.

Personality starts quite early in life. Fundamental differences in temperament are evident in human babies at the age of three or four months. This harks back to what I was talking about before in a previous lecture about infancy. That magic age of three months or so is when differences and capabilities start really becoming apparent in infants. What is going on here is that perhaps there is this genetic heritance that becomes apparent at three or four months. That infant temperament then provides a bias starting point for the development of personality over time and then a combination of innate mechanisms and individual experience then influences the eventual outcome of personality development.

It is true that parents can have relatively little influence on personality. But there is an interesting example and it serves as a bit of counter-example. This is interesting because it tells us a little bit about the biology of a personality trait, but it also tells us something about how it is possible, in certain cases, to influence personality. That example is reactivity. Reactivity is one of these personality traits. It is associated with an everyday phenomenon of shyness. One can study this in infants very easily, therefore I think the ease of studying it is probably why it is so often studied. The ease of studying is how infants react to unexpected objects or unexpected noises. It turns out that when you look at the reaction of infants to these unexpected objects or noises, about 15 percent to 20 percent of infants are high reactive. What that means is that they react with distress and they kick or cry when they are exposed to something new but not especially scary. For instance if you have a crib and you dangle a mobile over the crib, just the new mobile will evoke some kind of fear reaction, some kind of anxiety reaction, in 15 percent to 20 percent of babies for no apparent reason.

This high reactivity trait is retained for years. As these babies become toddlers, they tend to be what researchers call "behaviorally inhibited." Translating that into everyday English, what that means is that these kids are shy. High reactive babies, shy babies, tend to become introverted as toddlers and later. They are at higher risk than calm babies, the rest of the babies, of growing up to be worriers. These kids are more likely to become people who tend to spend a lot of time thinking about all the bad things that might happen to themselves or to their loved ones. Some fraction of people turn into this.

It turns out that about half of all high reactive babies become fearful children some time before age seven and then it declines over age. It turns out that only a third of them become obviously anxious adults. So this tendency diminishes. It is only in a minority of high reactive babies but some babies become anxious adults. It also turns out that high reactive babies also have a high risk of psychiatric anxiety disorders. Although low reactive babies also have some risk.

Let's get back to the topic of environmental influence. Let's ask the question, can this path be modified? One set of evidence comes from rats. It turns out that rat mothers who lick and groom their babies a lot produce offspring that are less timid and more prone to exploration than offspring of mothers who do less grooming. The same behavior outcome is seen in pups from low grooming mothers who are essentially adopted, raised by high grooming mothers. So being adopted by a high grooming a mother reduces anxiety.

Here is another example and this is an example closer to our species, rhesus monkeys. Like humans, about 20 percent of this species' young animals are high reactive. That is that they are stressed by unfamiliar situations that normal monkeys have no problem with. As in humans, this high reactive temperament in monkeys is highly heritable. You can look at monkeys and you can see biological mechanisms that correspond with reactivity, in particular, stress related signaling pathways which we now know about from a previous lecture.

When you take a high reactive monkey and you put that monkey in an unfamiliar playroom with new peers, they show physiological signs of stress. In particular, they show higher heart rates, higher blood levels of stress hormones such as ACTH and cortisol. They also show signaling differences in their fast response pathway, noradrenalin. Their noradrenalin metabolism turns over more quickly; noradrenalin is made and metabolized more quickly. That suggests that it cycles through the nervous system more quickly in high reactive monkeys.

It is also possible, in the face of all this biology, to affect the outcome of these high reactive monkey babies. It is possible to do it, specifically again, by parenting, by cross fostering. If you take a high reactive rhesus monkey baby and have it adopted by a calm mother, the high reactive babies who are placed with calm mothers are better at coping and avoiding stress as adults than similar young monkeys raised by reactive mothers. What is interesting that it does not go in the other direction. What is interesting is that monkeys who are not high reactive, young monkeys, do not show much effect, they do not care, basically, if they are cross fostered by a nurturing mother or an anxious mother. So it suggests that it is the high reactive monkeys that are vulnerable to variations in parenting quality. It is reminiscent of other findings in early development that basically the more important thing is to avoid deprivation as opposed to providing enrichment.

Finally, human infants who are unusually irritable at 15 days of age are more likely than other babies to become insecurely attached to their mothers at one year. But the outcome is much less likely if the mothers are trained in how to soothe restless babies.

To summarize this part then, it turns out that it appears that coping is a mechanism that can be taught or learned. Indeed it is generally observed that most children in the high reactive group, in fact, become successful. They learn how to deal constructively with their natural vigilance. Maybe they become interested in an activity that provides distraction from their worries along with positive reinforcement for their abilities, dance class, horseback riding, and math camp. Also, warm support of parents can encourage children to explore and engage with the world as long as they do not push so hard that they cause additional anxiety. So the action item here is that if your child is high reactive, then the situation can be handled by parental nurturing.

Finally I just want to make a brief note that personality is also changeable over life. This is true for octopuses. For instance, octopuses change in their personality from three weeks of life to six weeks of life, an aggressive animal can become shy and after that they become set in their ways. That is true in us as well. Humans are malleable in personality before the age of 30, then we become more stable. We are most stable of all when we get to the age range of 50 to 70. So human personality is malleable and then stabilizes.

To summarize what we have talked about today. Personality can be described by multiple dimensions, or clusters, in animals and in humans. Personality is something that is inheritable but caused by many genes, it is polygenic. Environmental influences are strong in influencing in personality but it is mostly not parental. It is something else in the environment. I have talked about an exception; the exception is shyness and anxiety. These are personality traits that are somewhat avoidable if you start early. Finally, as I said, personality is something that changes throughout life.

So we have talked about personality and its influences. Now what we will do in the next lecture is we will start talking about intelligence.

Intelligence, Genes, and Environment
Lecture 25

This excess brain, EQ, the amount of the brain occupied by forebrain, varies among species. It turns out that those variable proportions in particular are very predictive of problem solving and tool making.

This lecture discusses the genetics of intelligence and its environmental influences in terms of some controversial questions: Is it possible to increase the average intelligence of the population? Are there measurable differences between the sexes? Are there measurable differences between races? Can a finding be statistically significant yet have a small effect? What do averages and statistically significant differences tell us about individuals?

Quite early on, researchers observed that there is no correlation between brain size and intellectual accomplishments. Size difference has no direct correlation with performance. But interest in correlating brain size and biological factors with intelligence has been around for a long time—in particular, in the eugenics movement that took place between about 1900 and 1940. The hope of the eugenics proponents was to identify differences among groups and, perhaps, find ways to make the human race better. But group differences that are strong in one generation don't necessarily carry over into the next; thus, there is difficulty with the idea that a difference can be bred in the population.

Intelligence has multiple aspects, one of which is "fluid intelligence": the ability to reason through a problem you've never seen before. Fluid intelligence is correlated with working memory, which is the ability to hold information in your brain for several seconds, and with the ability to resist distractions. These capacities require the action of specific brain regions, some of which are in the **basal ganglia**. One is the striatum, a brain region that releases dopamine into parts of the frontal cortex; dopamine is both a reward signal and important in attention, in particular, for initiating and directing actions and thoughts and in updating information and working memory. Other regions important for fluid intelligence seem to be those with which the striatum communicates, particularly the prefrontal cortex, structures that seem important for resisting distraction.

The role of genetics in determining intelligence is complex and less well developed than the study of personality, but comparisons of identical twins with fraternal twins suggest that the prenatal environment appears to contribute about 20% of the variation in fluid intelligence. A key caveat here is that studies that show heritability of intelligence have been done in middle-class households with normal resources, without deprivation. This fact is critical because deprivation, as an environmental factor, is important in determining fluid intelligence. When the environment is bad, the influence of genes drops to as low as 10%. In general, the evidence points toward the conclusion that intelligence is predicted by both genetic and environmental factors. Under conditions of deprivation, environment wins. Under conditions of plenty, genes and environment seem to make approximately equal contributions.

But are fluid intelligence and problem solving really the right way to define intelligence? Objections to this definition include the idea that our brains have multiple capacities, such as emotional intelligence, the ability to read people's emotions and respond appropriately. Another objection is that test performance can be influenced by expectations, both external and internal. A third objection is a basic one: Tests only measure test-taking ability. All the consequences that come later in life, success and all the things we all know from everyday experience, don't necessarily correlate with fluid intelligence or any other kind of intelligence. ∎

Important Term

basal ganglia: A number of nuclei located subcortically in the forebrain. Many of the basal ganglia nuclei are involved in the extrapyramidal motor system.

1. Some people argue for the role of family life and genetics in determining intelligence, while others argue for the importance of resources, such as school funding. Considering the heritability of intelligence in normal and deprived environments, who is right? Are both right?

2. Describe a good pre-test strategy for maximizing performance on an exam.

Intelligence, Genes, and Environment
Lecture 25—Transcript

Welcome back. In the last lecture we examined how genes and environment worked together to determine personality. Now what I'd like to do is take the same approach, and take a similar arc, and apply it to a similar subject, although this subject is one that is more controversial. It's the subject of intelligence.

So for today what I want to do is talk about intelligence and its genetics and environmental influences. I want to couch it in terms of questions that you perhaps have run across, some of which are rather controversial. But I want you to think about these questions a little bit as we begin.

So one question that comes up a lot is, is it possible to breed humans to increase the average intelligence of the population? Another question that comes up in discussions, political discussions in particular, is, are there measurable differences between the sexes? Are there measurable differences between races?

Another question to think about is, can a finding be statistically significant yet have a small effect size, a small size that would not necessarily be easily observable in everyday life? A matching question to that is, what do averages and what do statistically- significant differences tell us about individuals?

So these are the questions I want us to start with and have in our minds as I present evidence to you today.

So in the study of intelligence, one basic question we can ask is, is it even possible to define intelligence? I mentioned the difficulties in defining personality in the previous lecture. Now let's apply that kind of critical examination to the subject of intelligence. We often hear about IQ, which is a single measure, a number that we can say that 100 is average, above 100 is above average, and so on. We also hear about multiple intelligences. So intelligence appears to be something that could be complex. Another question is, does intelligence change over life? Is it something that's trainable? These questions can be looked at both in humans and also in animals. What

I'd like to do is talk about that evidence first in animals and then move on to humans.

Firstly, can we look at intelligence in animals? It turns out that there are ways in which we can. Certain measures in intelligence in animals include social complexity, tool use, tool manufacturer, and what's called "proto-tool use," so using something, like for instance birds will use a crevice to break something. That is called "proto-tool use," and most generally problem solving. All these are things that we can measure in other animals.

It turns out that all these traits, problem solving, social complexity in building social networks, these traits are correlated with excess brain. Here's what I mean by excess brain. When you have a body of a certain size, when a species has a body of a typical size, the brain varies with that body size. So it turns out to be the case that larger bodies are associated with having larger brains. An elephant has a bigger brain than a mouse, obviously. But an elephant also has a bigger brain than a deer.

So there's a tendency for brain and body size to go together. But against that backdrop, there is also variation. That variation has been called a variety of things. One thing it has been called is "encephalization quotient," "EQ." Another way to measure the variation is that people have noticed that the biggest source of variation is how much of the brain is occupied by forebrains.

So for instance if you look in us and other mammals, the forebrain is dominated by the neocortex, the structure that we've talked about so much. If you look in birds, the forebrain is just forebrain. So it's the telencephalon. It doesn't have the same structure as the neocortex, and so one would not call it neocortex because it doesn't have that layered structure that we find in mammals.

This variation, this excess brain, EQ, the amount of the brain occupied by forebrain, varies among species. It turns out that those variable proportions in particular are very predictive of problem solving and tool making. So it appears to be the case that you can find a relationship between brain structure and measures of intelligence, problem solving in non-human species. So just right off the bat this seems kind of promising, the fact that we can see a relationship between the brain and intelligence. So this bodes well initially. However, it turns out that that's the good news for associated brain function with intelligence; the best information comes from comparisons among species.

It turns out that within species brain factors, brain anatomy, seems to be much less predicted. So it's much more difficult to come up with a correlation between brain proportions or brain size within a species. For example, if you look among humans, among individual humans, there's not very much variation in brain size. There is no difference in us that corresponds to the difference between, say, an elephant or a deer.

It turns out that what variation there is, is not very correlated with intelligence. So there's a famous example back in the 19th century, the story is described by Stephen J. Gould, the evolutionary biologist, in his book, *The Mismeasure of Man*. He describes a phenomenon back then in which great thinkers, for sport, gave their brains to be weighed after death. So they would donate their brains to be weighed. The question is asked, well, how big is this Englishman's brain? How big is this Frenchman's brain?

It turns out that from that time it was observed quite early on that there was not very much correlation between brain size and intellectual accomplishments. So it was possible to have a large brain or a small brain and yet have unpredictable influences on ideas. So there was a large variation in brain size even among accomplished people.

Another example is in the size difference between men and women. It turns out that men have larger brains than women. Even when accounting for body size, a man and a woman of similar body weight have different brain sizes. In fact men have brain sizes that are about 10 percent larger than women's on average. Yet men do not do better on intelligence tests on average. This is a case again in which there seems to be some size difference, but it doesn't have a direct correlation with performance. So there is difficulty already in looking for biological factors that influence intelligence.

Now I want to step back and ask the question of considering the idea that it's possible to influence intelligence genetically. It turns out that interest in brain size and intelligence, and biological factors and intelligence, has been around for a long time. In particular I want to spend a little bit of time talking about the Eugenics Movement.

Eugenics was big in the period of about 1900 to 1940. In fact as it turns out, modern statistics has its roots partly in efforts to identify differences among human groups. Statistical methods that we use today for other purposes come in part from that period of looking for genetic differences, looking for statistical differences, among groups. At that time mathematicians developed tools to quantify differences among groups. The hope at that time was an idealistic one. It was to find differences among groups and perhaps find ways to make the human race better. What's interesting here is that this was a hope that was held by very different political groups. Whether you were liberal, conservative, whatever your point of view was politically, it was nearly universal that people were interested in eugenic approaches to improving the human race.

What that means is it led to phenomena such as the proposal for selective breeding. It led to compulsory sterilization. It led to putting people on boxcars and sending them into prison camps.

It's possible to criticize eugenics on several grounds. Let's just bring up a moral criticism of eugenics. The moral criticism is that it's wrong to tell people to breed or to prevent them from doing so. That's an obvious criticism of eugenics. But what I want to do today is talk about the foundation of the idea, to talk about the science behind it, and consider whether this idea of eugenics is even well founded scientifically.

To start off with the problem, the basic problem with eugenics is that there are large environmental contributions to intelligence. What that means is that if there is a group difference between one group and another group of people, then group differences that are strong in one generation don't necessarily carry over into the next. So as a result there is a difficulty with the very idea that somehow a difference can be bred in the population.

In order to reach this conclusion what we have to do is we have to consider the various bits of evidence. I just want to outline where we're about to go here. I want to talk to you about how we define intelligence in the first place. I want to talk about what would constitute a large difference; whether those differences can be inherited, and what factors influence the inheritability of intelligence. I want to talk about what interventions seem to have a large effect on intelligence, whether it's even possible to take the converse to the eugenic point of view, what interventions can have an effect on intelligence.

First let's ask the question, can we define intelligence at all? So let's give it a try. We're going to talk about a factor called "g." Intelligence has multiple aspects. What we're going to do today is focus on fluid intelligence, which is what people typically mean when they talk about intelligence in modern times.

Fluid intelligence means the ability to reason through a problem you've never seen before. These problems typically take the form of logic puzzles, say for instance the dentist is sitting next to Mrs. E; Mrs. E is sitting next to a man; and the man is between two women; puzzles like that. These logic puzzles that require some amount of memory and logic to work through.

Different tests of intelligence, different aptitude tests, test for this kind of fluid intelligence to a different extent. It's possible to see this difference among different types of tests by looking at data gathered by James Flynn. Remember when we talked about development I talked about the Flynn Effect. This is an effect in which general performance in a variety of intelligence tests has increased over time.

So over a period of decades children and adults in many different countries, in developed countries, have done better on intelligence tests. So it's possible to look at data collected by Professor Flynn, and look at differences in different kinds of tests, and the way that they are related to this phenomenon of fluid intelligence.

For example, Professor Flynn has gathered information on factual knowledge, information on arithmetic and vocabulary. These are tests that don't test fluid intelligence. They test facts and just information that's retained. It turns out that since World War II the gain on those kinds of tests has only been a few IQ points, of typically five or fewer IQ points. So those are tests in which the Flynn Effect has not been seen.

Other tests have more requirements for fluid intelligence. So for instance if we look at things like block design, object assembly, arranging pictures, and organizing pictures, these are tests that seem to draw more on this phenomenon of fluid intelligence. It's possible to see increases of 15 to 20 points, and even higher, over that period of the end of World War II to now.

So those are tests that seem to be more dependent on this fluid intelligence capability. One of the best of all is something called "Raven's Progressive Matrices." This is a test in which you have a pattern, and you basically complete the pattern by showing patterns. It avoids vocabulary issues by using no words at all. This is a test in which people are shown a set of geometrical shapes with common characteristics, and then asked to choose another shape that fits into the set. This is a very interesting test because it appears to be most dependent, most related to, this phenomenon of fluid intelligence.

In general these different tests are referred to as having different amounts of g-loading. The term used by intelligence researchers is "g-loading." So a test that requires lots of fluid intelligence is more g-loaded. So for instance Raven's Progressive Matrices is more g-loaded than say picture completion or object assembly.

So now we've defined very carefully this one particular aspect of mental function, fluid intelligence. Now what I'd like to do is talk about what's known about neural substrates for intelligence. In other words, what parts of the brain are responsible for the activity of fluid intelligence for problem solving.

It turns out that brain regions that are involved in fluid intelligence also are involved in other abilities that seem to be related to fluid intelligence. So these particular capabilities are related to fluid intelligence and they seem to require a common set of brain regions. In particular, fluid intelligence is correlated with working memory. So working memory is a particular form of memory. It's the ability to hold information in your brain for tens of seconds. So if you remember a house number to go to a party, or if you remember a phone number to go dial it, that's working memory.

It turns out that intelligence is correlated with working memory. Intelligence is also correlated with the ability to resist distractions. So if you have things going on around you, if you temporarily turn your attention to something else and you're able to come back, that ability to direct your attention and resist distraction is also correlated with fluid intelligence.

Some of these capacities require the action of specific brain regions, some of which are in the core of the brain, in the basal ganglia in particular. One place that seems to be involved, for instance, in working memory is the striatum. The striatum is part of the basal ganglia. The striatum is a brain region that we've encountered before. It releases dopamine; and dopamine is a reward signal. Remember that dopamine is important in reward and attention. It seems to be important, in particular, for initiating and directing our actions and thoughts. This is a big function of the basal ganglia. The striatum in particular releases dopamine and releases it into parts of the frontal cortex. It seems to be important in updating information and working memory.

This is possible to see in brain scans, if you look at people who are involved in doing an updating task, you can see activity in the striatum. So an example of updating and working memory would be if you have working memory and you're trying to update the information. An example of updating is let's say you have a delivery route, and you're trying to get to the next three places, as you make your deliveries, the next three places you have to get to change. That's an example of updating. So remembering that running list of three places and being done with one and then moving onto the next one. That would be an example of updating. Updating is an activity that requires the striatum. The striatum is important in functions like that.

Other brain regions that are involved in fluid intelligence and also in working memory are of course in the neocortex, and in particular strong candidates for fluid intelligence substrates, are regions with which the striatum communicates. So the strongest candidate for the capacity of fluid intelligence is the prefrontal cortex. In particular, damage to the prefrontal cortex leads to difficulty with many forms of abstract reasoning and also working memory. So working memory requires the prefrontal cortex.

It has also been observed that there is a correlation, a weak correlation, between the volume of the prefrontal cortex and fluid intelligence. So when you look in a population of people you can find some relationship between prefrontal volume and fluid intelligence.

Another part of the cortex that's specifically related is part of the prefrontal cortex, the lateral prefrontal cortex. This is a part of the cortex that's activated by multiple different intelligence tests. So when you start going to the side, you can find brain regions in brain scanning, in fMRI studies, that are activated by multiple intelligence tests.

These are not the only regions. So for instance, parietal areas of cortex are also activated during many brain scanning studies of abstract reasoning and intelligence. These structures seem important for resisting distraction. It turns out that there's an interaction between the striatum, which I mentioned, and prefrontal and parietal activity. In particular, a lot of activity is seen in these cortical regions at high- distraction moments in persons with high fluid intelligence. It seems like these areas are quite active in people with high fluid intelligence.

If we put these together, what these ideas suggest is that there's a "fronto-striatal" network. A network involving frontal regions of the brain and also the striatum, in which different brain regions in or near the front of the brain are coordinated by the striatum and the action of dopamine.

What are the implications of this? Well, one implication is that working memory appears to be central to fluid intelligence. So maybe we could practice that. So it might be possible, for instance, to practice a working memory task and become better at one's fluid intelligence.

There is some evidence that practice at updating, this phenomenon with the three stops that I described, updating the list of three stops, can improve working memory. This touches upon the possibility that somehow fluid intelligence could be improved through practice at a working memory task.

This is a very active area of research. People are trying to find an association between working memory practice and fluid intelligence.

It turns out that there are challenges in designing such a good study. One of the challenges is in designing the thing that you practice to be sufficiently different from the fluid intelligence test that when you practice the task, you're not practicing the same task. So there are some challenges with designing a study to be done well. But I think that in the next few years it's likely that we are going to find out whether it's possible to improve fluid intelligence through a working memory practice task.

Again to continue a parallel structure to what we did when we talked about personality, now I want to talk about the role of genetics in determining intelligence. This turns out to be a complex subject. It's a subject that is less well developed than the study of personality. The method, at least in the initial stages, is the same.

The initial step is to look at similarity in different kinds of siblings. So if you look in humans, you can look in siblings who are non-twins, so regular siblings, or twins. The phenomenon that has been observed is that there's the largest amount of similarity in fluid intelligence in pairs of identical twins, and then less similarity in fraternal twins, and less similarity still in siblings. So it's siblings less than fraternal twins, less than identicals.

What this suggests is the following. Identical twins share of course both genes and a common pre-natal environment. What that means is that we can learn something about pre-natal environment by comparing identical twins and non-identical twins who share the pre-natal environment, but don't share as much genetic overlap. So identical twins as I said are more correlated than siblings, but less than identicals. These comparisons suggest that the pre-natal environment appears to contribute about 20 percent of the variations in fluid intelligence, so about a fifth of the variation in intelligence comes from the pre-natal environment.

If we look at the genetic aspect, the genetic aspect suggests that genes count for about 40 to 50 percent of the individual variability in general intelligence. So that is more, in fact, than the amount of influence on personality. So something like almost half of the variability in general intelligence appears to be connected with genetics.

A key caveat here is that these are studies that are done in middle-class households with normal resources, without deprivation. It turns out that studies that show heritability of intelligence come from middle-class households. The reason that I'm saying this is that the case of deprivation, as I've mentioned before, is very important. Environmental factors are quite important in determining fluid intelligence. By environmental factors, I mean education, nutrition, family environment, so we've talked about early development in the first three years of life; and also environmental features such as lead paint and the presence of other neurotoxins.

When the environment is bad, this influence of genes is not the same anymore. Instead of being half or almost half of the influence, the influence of genes drops to as low as 10 percent. So in the presence of a deprived environment, genetics has a very low influence on intelligence.

To summarize, genes seem to be involved in setting an upper limit on possible performance. Yet the range of environmental factors found in the United States and other developed countries can determine whether people reach that full genetic potential. So that's the bottom line for the genetics of intelligence.

Now let's take this back to a few points made in previous lectures. I've talked about topics relevant to this in a few ways. One is, think about neuroscience and think about the neuroscience in particular of early development. Remember I said that activity changes the brain during development in the form of neuroplasticity. In particular, external factors, especially deprivation, can influence development.

So this leads to several consequences which I've summarized already, and I've talked about already. One consequence appears to be the Flynn Effect. That effect is that IQ changes over time, over less than one generation, too fast for genetic selection. So this environmental influence can be seen there, in particular, probably relating to deprivation.

Another thing that I've told you about is early life environmental studies, so both correlative and also interventional studies. The finding is basically that parenting style in the first three years of life is correlated with IQ measured at the age of three. That's even true within a socioeconomic group. Furthermore, there's the finding that in deprived households, intervention in preschoolers leads to measurably better life outcomes at the age of 27.

So the general lesson from all of this, then, is that the evidence points towards the conclusion that intelligence is predicted by both genetic and environmental factors. Under conditions of deprivation, environment wins. Under conditions of non-deprivation, genes and environment seem to make approximately equal contributions.

So far that's the story, but it turns out that the story gets a little bit more complicated. For instance intelligence is not constant over life. Just as personality is somewhat variable, intelligence also varies as we get older. In fact, in particular when measured late in life, intelligence becomes more strongly predicted by genetics; that's interesting. It appears to be that our intelligence is not as correlated with genetics when we're younger, but becomes more correlated as we get older, which is funny. It's not clear why that is. One possibility for instance is that perhaps people seek out professions that reflect their genetic predispositions. Maybe you have a tendency to get into a thinking profession, so then you seek that out. Then that reinforces and drives you in the direction that's predicted by your genetics.

So to get it back to the eugenics movement, I would summarize the findings for that as follows. Even though the eugenics movement in many cases was well intentioned, and in some cases not, its scientific foundation was not very good. It had a poor scientific foundation. It turns out, given our current understanding, if the goal is to improve overall average intelligence in society, perhaps a more effective intervention would be to improve the environments of children who would not otherwise live to their genetic potential.

We spent all this time talking about fluid intelligence and problem solving. Perhaps one question that may be in your mind right now is whether that's really the right way to define intelligence. Remember that I went to a fair amount of effort to prescribe what I meant by "intelligence," in particular problem solving, and in particular Raven's Progressive Matrices.

One objection to this definition of intelligence is that there are multiple intelligences, our brains have multiple capacities. I gave you a fundamental piece of evidence of that. Remember I pointed out the case that different tests that I talked about had different amounts of g-loading. Even these different tests that Professor Flynn talked about have different amounts of g. G is not the only mental capacity. For example think about other capacities such as emotional intelligence, the ability to deal with people emotionally, to read their emotions and respond appropriately.

Emotional intelligence is a real and measurable capability. There are other kinds of intelligences that one can measure in people. These other kinds of intelligence are not the same as fluid problem-solving intelligence. So one objection to the things I've been talking about is that the focus has been on fluid intelligence, but there are other kinds of intelligence as well.

It is worth nothing that performance of these other areas is often correlated with fluid intelligence. So someone who has a lot of fluid intelligence tends to have more of these other intelligences. Not always, as we know from everyday life, but often it is the case that these capacities seem to vary together.

The point I'm trying to make is that there are other brain capacities besides fluid problem solving. Another objection to the idea of comparing intelligence and studying it in the way that I've described is that test performance can be influenced by expectations. Here's an area where knowing about this possible objection can influence our everyday lives. For example consider stereotypes, expectations that other people have of us. There's a famous study done by a colleague of mine at Princeton University, Professor Cecilia Rouse, looking at tryouts for European Symphony Orchestras. What she found was that tryouts used to be done in a way in which the jury could see the person trying out.

What she and a colleague did was a simple study in which they put a barrier up, and then it was not possible to see the person trying out. It turned out that the outcome was quite different gender wise. It turns out that if the jury could not see the auditioner, then many more women made it to the next stage of auditions than if they could see the person. So that's an example of stereotyping. In this case the stereotype is that only men can play well enough to be in the European Symphony. So that was an important finding.

It turns out that we also stereotype ourselves. We carry around ideas about ourselves individually and also about our group. For example if you give a math test and you ask women to write down their gender at the start of that test, women have a lower score if they write down their gender at the beginning of the test. On the other hand, if you ask women to think about somebody high achieving, having them think about a high-achieving women raises the score.

So for instance there's a study that has been done on Asian women. Asian women have two stereotypes they can draw on. One is that women are less good at math. The other stereotype is that Asians are good at math. Depending on which thing you ask them about, if you ask them about their sex or about their ethnic background, you can get a decrease or an increase in score depending on the question.

One practical consequence of this is that there is an external influence on test performance. It may be, in fact, helpful to visualize a very accomplished member of your group, whatever your group may be. If you visualize a very accomplished member of your group, then that can possibly have a small positive effect on test performance.

So the point then is that prior expectations are drawn from a variety of sources. We have sources of information that we draw on, including cultural biases of what a group is like in fact or in our perception, and basically from our statistical experience with groups. So our life experiences with groups lead us to expect something from a particular group. But it's important to emphasize that that expectation doesn't necessarily tell us about individuals. It's helpful to get away from these ways of thinking.

Third objection, and this is a basic objection. Tests only measure test taking. So despite the fact that these are well defined characteristics that once can go in and design in a laboratory and then apply to human subjects, it turns out that these tests don't necessarily correlate with later life outcomes. For example, just pick the next step that comes after tests, academic performance. Performance in college is not necessarily predicted by test scores. So for example, men do worse in college math classes than predicted by their test scores. But women do better than predicted by test scores. So there's a sex disparity in the outcomes from test scores when applied to the classrooms. That's not to mention real life. All the consequences that come later in life, life success and all the things that happen as we all know from everyday experience, don't necessarily correlate with fluid intelligence or any other kind of intelligence.

So let's summarize what we've learned today. I've told you that like personality, intelligence can be defined in animals and also in humans. Intelligence tests can measure many capacities. I've described to you many different kinds of intelligence, but focused in particular on fluid intelligence. Like personality, fluid intelligence is to an extent inherited. That's true under normal conditions. So under normal environmental conditions there's a strong inherited component to intelligence.

Under conditions of deprivation, intelligence is mostly environmentally determined. Such conditions exist in lower socioeconomic conditions in the United States. So there's an exception to the rule that intelligence is inherited.

Finally, I've told you about intelligence test performance and how intelligence test performance can be influenced by prior expectations on the part of the test taker.

In these last few lectures we've talked about individual differences, personality, and intelligence. Now what I'd like to do in the next lecture is talk about how we change in response to individual situations. In particular I would like to move onto the subject of emotion in the coming lectures.

The Weather in Your Brain—Emotions
Lecture 26

> Emotions are organized brain responses to events in the world around us. So basically, emotions are ways to organize or ways of dealing with information.

In some sense, we can think of emotions as a means our brains use to contain knowledge, accumulate it over evolutionary time, and organize it as strategies and responses to be passed on across generations. Emotions are organized brain responses to events in the world around us. They help us focus on critical information and motivate us to shape our behavior, get what we want and avoid what we fear, and move to a previous or desired state. Emotions also are critical in influencing decision-making.

Following Darwin's observations of animals, theories of emotion were propounded by William James, who said that we meet only a small fraction of our brain's potential, and Walter Cannon, a pioneer in understanding the fight-or-flight response.

William James and a Danish scientist named Carl Lange proposed a theory of emotion called the James-Lange theory, which suggested that we experience emotion in response to physiological changes and that those changes then change our perception of what we are feeling. James and Lange believed that those physiological changes were the emotion and that emotion consisted of a feedback loop in which the brain told the body what to do and the body told the brain what was going on.

However, Walter Cannon, the discoverer of "fight or flight," and another scientist named Philip Bard pointed out that in fact, there's a problem with the James-Lange theory: That is, emotional experience can occur independently of emotional expression. Furthermore, some physical reactions are associated with multiple emotional states. For example, both fear and anger are associated with an increased heart rate, inhibition of digestion, and increased sweating. A physical condition, such as a fever, can also lead to these reactions. Thus, it seems that fear cannot be purely a consequence of physiological changes. There must be something more to the story.

Different responses can share common neurotransmitters. Consider, for example, the adrenaline response. Adrenaline responses can be associated with different kinds of emotions, and to some extent, we can harness these emotions. For instance, if you get on a roller coaster, you get an adrenaline rush. Maybe you're afraid of it, or maybe you enjoy it. That same adrenaline rush can make the experience enjoyable or horrible.

The study of brain regions that are involved in emotional response goes back about 100 years. Broca noticed that there was a ring of structures around the **brain stem** that seemed different from the rest of the brain because of either their connections or their appearance. He called this area the "limbic lobe," "limbic" meaning peripheral region, or ring-like region. Papez, a later neurologist, suggested that there was an emotion system, a circuit of brain regions, many of which were collected near the midline in the brain, now called the **limbic system.** ■

Important Terms

brain stem: A phylogenetically older area of the brain consisting of the midbrain, metencephalon, and myelencephalon.

limbic system: A part of the brain most strikingly involved in emotion. Some major parts include the hippocampus, amygdala, hypothalamus, and septum.

Questions to Consider

1. What is the positive role of emotions in guiding action and decisions?

2. Compare the James-Lange theory of emotions with our expanded current understanding of how the brain and body influence emotional response.

The Weather in Your Brain—Emotions
Lecture 26—Transcript

Welcome back. In the last few lectures we've talked about individuality from the point of view of how we have individual personalities, how our intelligence may vary from individual to individual. Now what I'd like to do is I'd like to get into how we react to individual situations. In particular the next few lectures will concern the subject of emotion.

What I'd like to do is organize lectures into the following categories. We'll talk about emotion, and that's going to be the big emphasis in this lecture and the next lecture. Then we'll follow it with the discussion of mood. So we're really going to be starting the discussion of emotions; and really this lecture and the next lecture are quite intertwined. The topics will be first an overview today of emotions. Then we'll get into stronger emotions such as anger, fear, and anxiety.

As I talk about emotions, I want to again follow an arc that's similar to what I've talked about when I've talked about personality and intelligence, which is to start from animals as a way of beginning to understand what emotions are, and to look at the ancestral emotions that occur in all animals that are shared by us. I want to make a distinction between emotions and moods, what emotions are good for. I'll talk about biological and neural mechanisms of emotion. Then I'll spend some time talking about how we differ from other animals.

The study of emotion in animals and in humans has been around for almost two centuries. If we go back about 150 years we can see that there was interest in emotions in animals on the part of Charles Darwin. After he published the *Origin of Species*, he spent a lot of time researching the expression of emotions in man and animals, and wrote a book by that title, published in 1872.

At that time Darwin was very interested in the similarities in emotional expression between humans and animals. So what Darwin noticed time and again with angry faces, happy faces, sad faces, he noted similarities in emotional expression between humans and animals. He also noticed differences in say body postures, for instance in dogs and cats.

That was Darwin's work in the 19th century. He was primarily interested in the physical expression of the emotions, but he was not mainly focused on mental processes. It came to later researchers to spend specific efforts on the mental processes underlying emotions, not only how they're generated but also what they're good for.

Now researchers think of emotions as organized brain responses. So if we consider brain mechanisms of emotions, emotions are organized brain responses to events in the world around us. So basically emotions are ways to organize, or ways of dealing with information. They help us focus on critical information in the world around us, for instance say the threat of physical harm. So something imminent, bad may happen to us, and we focus on that. Or perhaps social opportunities, if we see somebody friendly, then we want to focus on that person. So emotions motivate us to shape our behavior. They help us get what we want. They help us avoid what we fear.

This is a general version of something I've talked about before in the context of stress. Remember in the context of stress I talked about allostatic response, the idea that the stress response is one that helps us get back to a prior state. I would present to you emotions as a means of moving an animal, including us, an animal or human, into a prior state, or to a desired state. So the idea that there's some state we're trying to get to, and emotions present a means of getting us towards that desired state.

Now I want to briefly contrast emotions with mood. Emotions are defined as a response to recent events. Mood refers to more of an overall emotional tone that's independent of momentary events. When I talk about mood later on and mood disorders, I'll talk about mood as opposed to emotions.

Emotions are critical in influencing our decision making. They're critical in living everyday life well. Remember when I talked about decision in a previous lecture, I talked about a famous patient who goes by the initials EVR. EVR had a tumor in the front of his brain. Remember he had surgery to remove the tumor, but that surgery also took out a big piece of part of his cortex around the orbit of his eye, the orbital frontal cortex.

After this surgery, EVR was still able to talk sensibly about the economy, foreign affairs, current events. He could solve complicated financial, ethical problems that were presented to him in the abstract. His memory and intelligence were unchanged. But he had trouble with minor decisions, big decisions. He just couldn't make decisions. He couldn't pick a shirt to wear in the morning. He lost his job. He was divorced by his wife. He went into bad business ventures, went bankrupt. He eventually moved in with his parents. Recall that I said he married a prostitute and was divorced again after six months.

What the case of EVR tells us is several things. The first thing it tells us is that evidently the orbital frontal cortex is involved with decision making. The second thing is that emotions are in particular absolutely necessary for good decision making. EVR was a man who was still able to experience emotions, but he had difficulty monitoring his own behavior. He had difficulty matching his behavior to the rules of social interaction. He had difficulty linking his emotional responses with cognitive decision making. So he was unable to connect his emotional reactions to situations with what he knew that he ought to do. He just couldn't do it.

Now I want to talk a little bit generally about this critical relationship between emotions and decision making. This relationship is understood to be very important. It's increasingly of interest in areas outside of neuroscience. So for instance, computer designers, people who work in artificial intelligence, have had some difficulties making machines that are good at decision making. It's difficult to get a machine to value one good as being greater than another good.

One trend in artificial intelligence is to build in affective responses, by which I mean emotional responses. So the idea is that value is place on outcomes, and that value is then something that guides the computer's responses. So emotions have, in some sense, started to play a role in the development of technologies in artificial thinking machines.

Another way to think about emotions and decisions and life is that emotions are a way for strategies and responses to be passed on. For instance, a set of responses to a particular situation, like a dangerous situation or a benign situation, tend to go together. So emotions are a way for us to organize, for our brains to organize, our responses to events. In some sense you can think of it as being like memories. Remember I talked about memory as being a way of learning about events that happened to us in our lives, and then save that for the future. Emotions also are a means of organizing our brain's responses. Except in the case of emotions, that way of organizing responses can be passed across generations.

So in some sense we can think of emotions as a means of our brain containing knowledge and accumulating that knowledge over evolutionary time. So that's one way to think about what emotions are.

I've introduced the subject of emotion, in particular this fellow EVR. Now I want to talk a little bit more about theories of emotion. I want to go back and take up the story just after Darwin and think about what it is that emotions are, and exactly how emotions are generated.

It turns out that several core theories of what emotions were propounded by people we've encountered already. We've encountered William James, who I said that he said that we only need a small fraction of our brain's potential, and also Walter Cannon. Remember when I talked about stress, Cannon was a pioneer in understanding the fight or flight response. So these two scientists also played a role in understanding emotion. They and others who I will name were involved in thinking about what emotions are and how they arise and what they're good for. In particular I'll start by talking about William James.

William James did his work mostly in the 19th century, a little bit in the 20th century. He and a Danish scientist named Carl Lange proposed a theory of emotion that's called "the James Lange theory." The two of them suggested the following model for how we experience emotions.

What James and Lange suggested is that we experience emotion in response to physiological changes. In other words you might imagine that we cry because we feel sad. What James and Lange thought was the converse. What they suggested was no, we actually feel sad because we cry. In particular, one can imagine a little causal diagram as follows. We can imagine a chain of events as proposed by James and Lange as follows.

Imagine a situation that you encounter, say a sad situation, and that situation causes sensory signals to be generated. Those sensory signals go to your brain. Then your brain takes those signals and sends commands out to the body. Those commands can take the form of, say, the sympathetic response, for instance changes in muscle tone and in heart rate. Other changes can go out to the body, including say crying.

What James and Lange suggested was that those changes then came back into the brain and changed your perception of what you were feeling. What they believed was that those physiological changes were the emotion and that those physiological changes then came back and fed back into the brain. So they basically believed that emotion consisted of a feedback loop in which the brain told the body what to do, and the body told the brain what was going on. That feedback loop was a key loop that began with the brain and critically involved the body.

So an example of this can be found in the case of blushing. So for instance let's think about blushing for a moment. There's a very good story that goes with this. If we think about blushing, blushing produces secondary effects. Blushing is embarrassing. It can cause intense self-consciousness, confusion, and loss of focus. In fact it is possible to induce blushing. So when I teach students I've done this where I take a member of the class and I point at him or her, and I just point at him or her. And I just say, okay, I'm pointing at you. And I make it clear at the beginning that I'm pointing for no reason at all. It's possible to induce blushing in that person, even though the person has done nothing. Yet, he or she begins to blush and starts to feel embarrassed, simply from me doing that. You can try this if you're speaking to a group sometime.

So let's think about blushing some more and its role in generating emotions. In this case I've talked about blushing as generating embarrassment. There's a very interesting case of an aspiring newscaster. This is a story that's described by Atul Gawande, the medical writer. Dr. Gawande has written a book of essays, collected from his various magazine articles, called *Complications*. He wrote an essay called, *Crimson Tide*. *Crimson Tide* concerns the story of a woman who's an aspiring newscaster named Christine Drury.

Christine Drury was ambitious. She wanted to become an anchorwoman for a TV station. And in 1997 she was 26 years old. She became the overnight anchorwoman at this TV station. It was an NBC affiliate, Channel 13 in Indianapolis. It turns out that being an overnight anchorwoman is, in fact, a stepping stone to being a daytime anchor. She wanted to do that. Her goal was to work up to being a daytime anchor. This was her ambition.

But she had a problem. Her problem was that she blushed very easily. When she did blush, she blushed uncontrollably. So for example if she stumbled on a word, she would blush. If she was standing in line at the store, if a grocery checker held up her cereal and said, I need a price on corn flakes over here, then she would in fact blush uncontrollably at the fact of a grocery checker calling attention to her.

So this is a funny disability in somebody who wants to be a TV newscaster, but it was a problem that she had. What's interesting is that in many ways she was a very social and gregarious person. In school she was a cheerleader. She was on the prom queen court. She was on the tennis team. She was a social, social person, and had in some ways very few problems in dealing with other people.

But she had this problem that she blushed. Getting back to Walter Cannon, I mentioned Cannon as a key player in theories of emotions. Cannon, remember, is a pioneer in outlining the sympathetic nervous system, the fight-flight response. The mechanism of blushing is part of the sympathetic nervous system. So recall that I told you about adrenaline being secreted by the adrenal gland, and then being sent to various organs around the body leading to changes to pupil dilation, the rate of the heart, digestion, and other parts of the body.

So blushing is part of that sympathetic nervous system. Blood gets sent into the face. That's part of blushing. Drury wanted to do something about her uncontrollable blushing. And she chose to have a technique done called "ETS." "ETS" stands for Endoscopic Thoracic Sympathectomy. Endoscopic surgery where a little slit is made, and then a surgeon goes in to the thorax, thoracic sympathectomy, cutting of the sympathetic nervous system.

Drury wanted this treatment, and she with her father traveled to Goteborg, Sweden, where there's an expert in this treatment. She had a Swedish surgeon go in and cut a part of her sympathetic nervous system, to cut a trunk of her sympathetic nervous system so that she would no longer blush.

It turns out that a number of things happened, so she lost other sympathetic nervous responses as well. She tended to not sweat nearly so much in her palms. She sweated more in her trunk. So there were other things that came with this sympathectomy. But one thing that was interesting was that she lost the blushing response, and she also lost self-consciousness. So there are several things that happened to her.

One thing that happened that was quite striking was right after her surgery an attractive male nurse came to take her blood pressure. This handsome guy came in to take her blood pressure. Normally she would have blushed, no problem. She was fine.

Later when she returned to work she recorded a TV segment of a bunch of eight-year-olds. These eight-year-olds were throwing things at the camera. They were just generally being disruptive. It was chaos. But throughout that segment she was able to remain composed, and she didn't blush. These are situations that previously would have caused her a great problem. So she lost her self-consciousness in response to the fact that she had had her sympathetic response cut.

That's interesting because it suggests it's at least consistent with the James Lange idea that our bodies, in this case her face, tell us something about our emotional state. That supports the case.

However, Walter Cannon himself, the discoverer of fight-or-flight, and another scientist named Philip Bard, pointed out that in fact there's a problem with the idea. The problem they pointed out is that emotional experience can also occur independently of emotional expression. So for instance they described an experiment in which an animal's spinal cord was transected. What that left was just an upper body and head able to respond. What they pointed out was that signs of emotion could still be expressed in the upper body of an animal even when it was not getting information from the lower body.

Another example they came up with was they pointed out the fact that some physical reactions are associated with multiple emotional states. So let's just talk about fear. We'll be coming back to fear in the next lecture. Fear is associated with an increased heart rate. It's associated with inhibition of digestion. It's associated with increased sweating. These are a few of the things I mentioned in the case of Christine Drury.

Anger also includes increased heart rate, inhibited digestion, and an increased sweating. So these are two very different emotions that both include some of the same physiological signs.

Furthermore, a non-emotional condition can also lead to these changes. In particular when we are ill, fever will also lead to these changes. People who are feverish are not particularly known for being fearful or angry. So what seems to be the case is that fear cannot be purely a consequence of physiological changes. There has to be something more to the story than physiological changes in determining emotion.

In fact again we can come back to the Christine Drury and we can look at her case. I told you that she did quite well with a TV segment shortly after her surgery. It turns out that six months later, her self-consciousness had returned. She started to feel uneasy. In fact some time after her surgery, she came out to a colleague, went out to dinner and said, and told the friend what she had done, that she had the sympathectomy. The friend was actually horrified that she would go to such lengths to further her career. So she became anxious that she was a fake. She started feeling self-conscious when she was on camera, and she had to quit.

She later did go back to work, but one of the things she did along the way is she went back and did radio work, where the blushing thing is not really a major factor. She didn't have to worry about the fact that she didn't blush.

Getting back to Cannon and Bard's suggestion that there has to be something more than this feedback from the body to the brain. Different responses can share common neurotransmitters. So if we think about the biological mechanism, think about the adrenaline response.

Adrenaline responses can be associated with different kinds of emotions, and to some extent we can harness these emotions. So for instance if you get on a roller coaster you get an adrenaline rush. Maybe you're afraid of it, or maybe you enjoy it. That same adrenaline rush can make the experience enjoyable or horrible.

Another example is public speaking. People are often afraid of public speaking. Public speaking is often considered a horrible experience in which one has some kind of sympathetic response in which one gets an adrenaline rush, and here I am in front of this crowd of people, and I feel a little bit afraid. It's possible to harness that feeling, to take that feeling that you get when you're in front of a group, and to harness that feeling to excitement to direct energies. And this is something that I've noticed for myself that I've been very interested in over time as I get used to speaking to large groups of people.

We've talked about animals. We've talked about humans. Now what I want to do is I want to spend some time talking about the biological mechanisms, the neural mechanisms, by which the brain produces and perceives emotions. Many of these mechanisms are shared with other animals. So I want to talk about that a little bit.

The study of brain regions that are involved in emotional response goes back about 100 years. Those ideas have been modified over time. Some of these ideas are not exactly right. But it's worthwhile to think about them a little bit.

If we go back to the neurologist, Broca, I've talked about Broca before because he's described Broca's brain area for language. Broca looked at a lot of brains during his career. One thing that Broca noticed was that there was a ring of structures around the brain stem. So the brain stem is at the core of the brain, and the neocortex and other forebrain structures are sort of up here. What he noticed was a ring of structures around the brain stem that seemed different from the rest of the brain due to either their connections or to their appearance.

He called this the "limbic lobe," "limbic" meaning peripheral region, or ring-like region. So Broca defined the limbic lobe. Papez, a later neurologist, proposed an emotion system. What Papez suggested was that there was an emotion system that linked the neocortex, this outer part, with the hypothalamus, this part of the brain that sits below the thalamus.

What Papez suggested was that there was a circuit of brain regions, many of which were collected near the midline in the brain, so near the middle plane of the brain. He suggested the circuit of brain regions, and it's even now called "the Papez circuit."

Today this Papez circuit is now called "the limbic system." It includes a number of regions. It includes the singulate gyrus. It includes, I mentioned it before, the anterior singulate. It includes the hypothalamus, the anterior thalamus, and the hippocampus. These are regions that are considered part of the limbic system.

Now this is not quite exactly the set of brain regions involved in emotion processing; but key regions are included there. So I describe it because some of these regions are known now to be critical in emotional processing. What I want to do is start from that description of the limbic system and broaden it to include other brain substrates of emotion that, in fact, are now understood to be very interesting parts of the brain's emotional response.

I've already talked previously about the anterior singulate cortex and prefrontal cortex. I've talked for instance about emotional responses in this fellow, EVR. In the next lecture I'm going to talk about some brain regions. I'm going to put them off for a little bit, in particular the hypothalamus, underneath the thalamus, and the amygdala. I'm going to have a lot to say about these because they play a wide range of functions in emotions. So I'm going to be talking about the hypothalamus and amygdala when I talk about anger, rage, fear, and anxiety.

What I want to do next, right now what I'd like to do is talk about the basal ganglia and the insular cortex. The insular cortex is a part of the cortex that's buried, and this part of the cortex that's sort of buried. It's not too far from some of these other regions that I've talked about. It also goes by the name of the "insula." This insula appears to be, along with the basal ganglia, key players in a certain emotion; that emotion is disgust. So I want to talk about disgust a little bit.

Disgust is an evolutionarily old mechanism. It's an old emotion. It dates back to the need for foraging animals to determine whether the food is good to eat. So whenever an animal is looking for something, is it good to eat? Is it not good to eat?

So disgust is something that's a critical emotional response. It's also an old emotional response. You can see disgust when you look at animals when they encounter a bitter or disagreeable substance. So for instance rats can make disgusted faces, "Ah, Ah." So rats will make faces when they encounter something not tasty.

Studies have been done on newborn rabbits. Newborn rabbits react differently when they encounter either a sweet or bitter solution. For instance if they encounter something bitter, they gape and turn their heads away. That's an expression of disgust. As opposed to encountering something sweet where they just engage in quiet licking. So if you give a rabbit something sweet to taste, it will just lick it quietly.

Key brain regions for generating these feelings of disgust, as I said, are the basal ganglia and the insula. In fact you can see evidence for this in animals and in humans. So for example, when the insula in humans is electrically stimulated, what are generated are sensations of nausea and unpleasant tastes. Remember that brain surgery is often done on awake patients in order to find out whether it's going to be bad to cut out a part of the brain. In some of these surgeries you can, in fact, see sensations of nausea and unpleasantness generated by stimulating the insula.

If you look in rats, if rats are damaged either in the basal ganglia or the insula, rats with damage to either of these areas have difficulty learning to avoid foods that make them sick. They're not good at determining what makes them sick.

In people, a wrinkle to this is that the role of these regions has been brought so that it's not only recognizing these feelings in ourselves, but in people, these brain regions also light up in brain scans when we see these feelings in other people. So these brain regions specifically light up when we notice the feeling of nausea or disgust in another person.

That's interesting, because what it shows is something a little bit more general, which is that patients with damage to the insula or the basal ganglia have difficulty recognizing facial expressions of disgust. Interestingly it's a side effect, it's a consequence, of Huntington's Disease. Huntington's Disease is a primarily motor disorder. It's caused by degeneration of neurons in the striatum, which is part of the basal ganglia. People with Huntington's Disease also have this difficulty.

There's other evidence as well, and I'll just summarize the other evidence. The other evidence taken together about what the insula does, is that the insula seems to be important not only with disgust, but more generally it seems to be important in decisions and social behavior. In particular, it seems to be important in regulating social behavior. It sends information to other areas involved in decision making. Remember I've talked about the emotion of decision making.

It turns out the insula sends information to the anterior singulate cortex and the prefrontal cortex. So it sends projections to frontal parts of the brain that seem to be important for social based decision making.

The insula seems in general to be important in regulating social behavior. So for instance it helps us infer emotional states, such as embarrassment, from looking at physical states such as a flushed face. The insula is one of several brain systems that responds in a similar way to our own actions or our own states, and those of another person. So the idea that we can see disgust in another person, and we can feel that disgust, and it leads to activation of our insula.

Remember I also mentioned the mirror neuron system in a previous lecture in which there are neurons that seem to be responsive to both acts of others and ourselves. So there are brain systems that do this. I'm going to be talking about these systems a little bit more when we talk about the social brain.

Now I want to broaden this even further. So I've talked about disgust. I've talked about emotional responses. I want to broaden this to not only physical disgust at something like rotting food. It turns out that these same brain regions that cause us to wrinkle our noses at spoiled food also cause us to recoil from moral decency. So when we encounter a situation that is morally repellant to us, this also makes our insulas light up. So the thought of a morally repulsive act leads our insula to light up.

In fact, getting back to the whole mirror idea, the insula is also active when people think about experiences that make them feel guilt. You can think of guilt as an emotion that in some sense is disgust that's directed toward oneself. So that feeling of guilt also lights up the insula, also causes activation of the insula.

This is interesting because one question that philosophers have asked is, where does the emotion and where does the cognitive process of moral disgust come from? This is something that philosophers have pondered. One way to think about it now that I've told you these facts about disgust is that if you think about what animals are capable of doing, animals are able to feel disgust at rotting food. So from an evolutionary standpoint, disgust is the older phenomenon. So disgust is something general among animals.

In us, we have a moral system. That new system, relatively new evolutionarily, takes advantage of this older existing brain function. So in some sense what we have here is a system of the brain whose job it is to register disgust. Our moral system is able to take advantage of that older function and use it to read out moral disgust.

Now let's review the insula a little bit. The insula's general job seems to be to sense the state of your body and trigger emotions that will motivate you to do what your body needs. It also turns out to also light up when you think you need something. So for instance, if you think you need something, an example of activation of the insula occurs when people crave nicotine and other drugs. It turns out that craving for drugs also lights up the insula. So these are all examples of the insula reporting states of things that our bodies need.

So far I've talked about mechanisms that are mostly shared between us and other animals, mechanisms that are rooted in our history as mammals, or as even vertebrates. Now what I'd like to do is I'd like to talk about emotional mechanisms that seem to differ between us and other animals.

I want to specifically focus on that. As I've mentioned before, a major difference between us and other animals is the fact that we have a lot of cortex. In particular we have a lot of frontal cortex. That size of the cortex has a consequence. The consequence is that human emotions seem to be more complex because of frontal influences on emotional response.

If you look at connections within the brain, it appears to be that frontal regions seem to inhibit the emotional system. So there's this inhibition that comes from frontal regions of the brain and inhibits emotional brain circuits. So what that means is that there are mechanisms for regulating social behavior, these emotions that control our social behaviors.

Many brain regions are important for emotion, and they also control social signals. So there is this interaction between frontal regions in evaluating situations and the emotional system. There's a lot of prefrontal control over emotions. There, correspondingly, are ways that emotional reactions can be modulated. I'll give you two examples.

One example is the phenomenon of distraction. For instance it's possible to decrease the negative emotions associated with physical pain by redirecting attention. If you are experiencing pain, you recall I talked about pain in a previous lecture, that perception of pain can be altered by turning one's attention away.

Conversely, it's possible to increase the feeling of pain or increase the intensity of an emotional response in general by focusing attention on that response. Remember I gave the example of a toddler whose subjective feeling of pain appears to be regulated by whether Mom is around or not. So distraction is a major component in regulating emotional response.

Another example of something that is well developed in us, in our species, is reappraisal. "Reappraisal" is defined as reconsideration of the meaning of an event. So for instance let's now consider that same child who experienced pain, let's say the kid touches a hot stove. Now let's consider how a parent, how I react, to her touching the hot stove. So maybe early on I might have an angry reaction. My angry reaction is, she disobeyed me and she touched the stove. So that would be a momentary reaction.

Then that might be replaced by guilt. I was not paying attention, and I let her touch the stove. It's my fault, and I feel guilty. Eventually, I might reappraise my reaction one more time. I might eventually feel less upset by thinking, well, she didn't injure herself too badly this time. The good news is that she has now learned to avoid a stove. So maybe it's going to be okay after all. That's an example of reappraisal.

Here's another example of reappraisal. You're about to meet your date at a restaurant. You're excited about meeting this person and that person is late. Your initial reaction might be one of anger, where were you? You are late for dinner, and I've been waiting here for an hour. If you find out that that person is late because he or she was helping somebody who had a heart attack, your feelings might be reappraised and you might shift to happiness and pride. Assuming that you believe the story that they were helping somebody with a heart attack, then you would perhaps reappraise.

One phenomenon that comes with reappraisal is that when people are studied in a scanner and examined, it turns out that their emotional regions involved in the emotional response that become less active, and in particular the amygdala becomes less active when people reappraise the situation. So that's something that's been seen in reappraisal, done by people in the scanner.

People who are good at reappraisal turn out to be emotionally stable and resilient. This reappraisal process seems to again involve prefrontal and interior singulate cortex, these frontal brain regions. What's interesting is that these same brain regions are all also activated when we take a placebo drug. So there seems to be something about regulating our response.

The lesson here is that reappraisal is a useful life skill. In particular I should point out at this point that reappraisal, getting back to something I talked about in the aging lecture, reappraisal is something that improves as we get older.

So let's summarize what we've learned today. We've learned that emotions guide reactions and decisions, a these emotions are central to survival. Referring back to the idea of allostasus, emotions are part of our allostatic response.

Many brain regions are involved in our emotional responses. They include the amygdala, the insula, the basal ganglia, and the singulate cortex. These are parts of the limbic system.

Some of these regions are involved in decision making and in moral judgments

and in social judgments. So these emotional responses are critical to a wide variety of daily functions. I have finally told you about emotional responses and how they're modulated by cognitive mechanisms.

In this lecture I've talked about emotion in general, and the context of how emotions guide our lives. In the next lecture what I would like to do is focus on certain strong negative emotions. In particular I would like to focus on anger, fear, and anxiety.

Fear, Loathing, and Anger
Lecture 27

> The hypothalamus is small; it's about the size of a large grape. It's less than 1% of the total volume of the human brain. Yet ... one can find all kinds of things packed within this very small structure.

Negative and very strong emotions are among those that regulate our behavior. Anger, fear, and anxiety originate in key brain structures that play a critical role in regulating strong emotions—the hypothalamus and the amygdala.

The hypothalamus, a central regulator of many of our most basic impulses, is less than 1% of the total volume of the human brain, yet it contains functions related to self-regulation and general emotional responses. It is a brain region, so its neurons send out axons, and it acts as a gland, so it secretes molecular signals in the form of hormones. These hormones coordinate the brain's and body's responses.

The amygdala can have a powerful suppressive effect on aggression, and it, too, seems to play a key role in driving strong emotional responses.

Let's just imagine for a moment that it's winter and that you're out hiking. You've been hiking a long way, and you're cold, dehydrated, low on energy. The hypothalamus takes signals from your viscera and your blood; processes them to make decisions about what to do; and starts sending signals about what should happen next. It will urge you to seek warmth, start moving around, drink water, and find some food.

The hypothalamus can also drive you powerfully to very intense responses. Experiments involving cutting into the brain and either leaving the hypothalamus attached to the brain stem or cutting it off from the brain stem have suggested that the hypothalamus plays a critical, necessary role for generating and controlling rage.

The amygdala can have a powerful suppressive effect on aggression, and it, too, seems to play a key role in driving strong emotional responses. It also organizes our responses to a possible danger stimulus, mediated by a rapid response from the visual system, and it can reduce physical signs of anxiety, such as sweating. This suggests that the amygdala is important in generating responses associated with fear.

The amygdala is also important in learning. A particular type of learning that involves fear conditioning has been studied in animals. It is possible to teach an animal, in a single trial, to be afraid of a neutral stimulus. But once learned, can fear memory be unlearned? It turns out that unlearning is much harder than learning in this case. Fear conditioning, evolutionarily, *must* be learned on a single trial because you might not get a second chance. Unlearning, however, requires many trials, and it seems to involve other structures, including the hippocampus and the neocortex.

Anxiety is closely related to fear. It is expressed in response to perceived danger as opposed to a specific event, such as whether we left the stove on when we left the house. The fear and anxiety system can malfunction to cause anxiety disorders, which can be debilitating. In anxiety disorders, the hypothalamic pituitary adrenal axis, the same axis involved in stress, shows a high level of activity. Anxiety disorders are marked by biochemical and neurological changes that are specific to the disorders, and one major hypothesis of anxiety disorder is that the axis malfunctions. It has been observed that maternal stress and the secretion of stress hormones are associated with later emotional problems, including anxiety disorders. This suggests that extreme stress in the mother can affect fetal brain development to influence the likelihood of an anxiety disorder. ■

Questions to Consider

1. What is the difference between homeostasis and allostasis?

2. What are the allostatic roles of emotion and stress?

Fear, Loathing, and Anger
Lecture 27—Transcript

Welcome back. In the last lecture we talked about emotion and we discussed, in general, its critical role in organizing our behavior and our decisions in everyday life, our reactions and ways in which emotion brings us back to some desired state of being. Now what I'd like to do is to continue that theme today and focus now on negative emotions and very strong emotions, and these are among the strongest emotions that regulate our behavior, powerful emotions. The ones I want to specifically focus on are anger, fear, and anxiety. I'm using these emotions as a way of focusing on key brain structures that play a critical role in regulating these strong emotions, and also some positive emotions as well. Those brain structures are the hypothalamus and the amygdala, and these brain structures play a critical role in generating anger and fear responses, and also in the case of amygdala, can change and lead to the learning of fear. So these are brain structures that I'm going to be focused on, and as I said, focusing on positive emotions as well.

Let's start with the hypothalamus. The hypothalamus is a central regulator of many of our most basic impulses. The hypothalamus is a structure that we've encountered before when we talked about the stress response, and recall the hypothalamus pituitary adrenal axis. One thing that part of the hypothalamus does is control the stress response. It turns out that the hypothalamus has many other jobs too. It plays many, many roles. It's the size of about a large grape, but within that large grape is carried many, many jobs. It mostly has the job of, very generally speaking, keeping us in balance, but occasionally does things that drive us very, very far from balance, very far from the even keel.

As I've said, the hypothalamus is small, it's about the size of a large grape. It's less than 1 percent of the total volume of the human brain. Yet within this small volume are packed many functions relating to self regulation, relating to general emotional responses, and one can find all kinds of things packed within this very small structure. Within the structure it's possible for the hypothalamus to regulate different responses separately. So it's very dense. One can think of it as basically the Grand Central Station of allostatic response and emotion.

The way that the hypothalamus does this is that it can send signals several different ways. The hypothalamic neurons, neurons of the hypothalamus, send axons out, and also the hypothalamus secretes molecular signals in the form of hormones. What that means is that in addition to being a brain region, it's got a special capacity relative to other brain regions, it acts as a gland. It secretes hormones into the fluid around it that then diffuse and act. These hormones coordinate the brain and body's responses in many, many arenas. We've talked about stress in a previous lecture, but also the hypothalamus regulates other functions that have to do with keeping us on an even keel and also regulating our response. I'll give you some examples, some early discoveries about the hypothalamus.

Many of the earlier discoveries of the hypothalamus were made by putting an electrode into a laboratory animal and stimulating to see what the animal did, and so experimenters had to put in a probe and look for this very small structure which is very, very small in a rat. The kind of thing they found out was that they could get really interesting responses by stimulating at different locations in the thalamus, just by moving around a little bit in this very tiny structure. One example is that stimulation of part of the thalamus seems to be rewarding. It seems to convey something like pleasure, and the way that they knew this was that a rat would run around the cage, and then the experimenters would stimulate the electrode and then the rats would tend to come back to the same part of the cage where the stimulation occurred. So they would make an association between some part of the cage and the activation of the hypothalamus, and they'd come back to say, well I want some more of that, whatever it is, and they would come back to that same part of the cage. So that's an example of one of the things that the hypothalamus seems to signal.

I want to now talk about a few things that the hypothalamus might do all at once, and I want to give you an example. Let's just imagine for a moment that it's winter and that you're out hiking. You're out there hiking, you've been hiking a long way, and you're cold, you're dehydrated, you're low on energy. It is time for your hypothalamus to do things. So what the hypothalamus does in this case is take signals from your body, from your viscera, and from your blood, and it takes those signals and it processes them to make decisions about what to do. It starts sending signals about what it is that should happen next. It sends signals that range from long-term signals to get you back on an even keel on a long-time scale, and also does immediate things. So the long-term signals, relatively long term, are the hypothalamus sends signals to make you shiver, to get you to warm up a little bit. It will send signals to redirect blood flow to go to the core of the body so you can preserve heat. Because you're dehydrated, it will send signals that inhibit the production of urine. Because you're low on energy, it'll send signals to mobilize body fat. It'll do all those things when you're cold, but all of those responses take time, and so those are ways in which the hypothalamus can help you get on an even keel on a long timescale, say hours. But the hypothalamus also triggers fast changes. It can get you to do things in response to these events of being cold and being thirsty and hungry. The hypothalamus will create in you urges, and you will go do these things. You will go seek warmth, you'll start moving around to try to warm up. You're thirsty, you will go drink water in response to these same signals. You're hungry, you're going to go find some food. You will start eating.

To summarize from this example, the hypothalamus is, in all these cases on this cold hike, the hypothalamus is trying to get you back to where you were. Like the stress response, these are examples of homeostatic regulation. Again getting back to the homeostatic and allostatic concept, the concept is that your body has some desired state. What the hypothalamus does in general in many cases is it integrates information from brain and body inputs and it figures out what it should take to get you back to your desired state, back to some starting state. Then it does things to direct you to go do that. That's, in a nutshell, one major role of the hypothalamus.

However, the hypothalamus can do much more than get you to where you were. It can also drive you powerfully to very intense responses. Some of these responses can propel us beyond simple homeostasis. They can direct us towards a major goal. They can make us do big, big things, in addition to just getting us back to where we were. So here I'll give an example, another example.

Here's an experiment that has been done on cats and also on rats, and it again involves sticking an electrode into the hypothalamus to find out what various parts of the hypothalamus do. It turns out that stimulation of one part of the hypothalamus leads to rage. What happens is that if you do this to, for instance, a cat, a cat with this particular part of the hypothalamus activated will attack a nearby animal or will just exhibit incoherent rage, arch its back, start hissing and spitting, and its fur will stand up. As soon as the stimulation ends—and by the way, these responses in fact also happen when there's no other animal present, so a cat will simply start doing this when this part of the hypothalamus is activated. When the stimulation ends the cat calms down immediately, and in fact, the cat will sometimes almost immediately just go right to sleep because as we all know, cats spend a lot of their time sleeping. This is the phenomenon of sham rage. That's the technical term for it. It's this phenomenon where activation leads an animal to act as if it's enraged and then the rage goes away as soon as the stimulation stops.

There's other evidence that sham rage is under control of the rest of the brain and this is work done by Philip Bard who we met in the last lecture. Bard did studies to find out exactly what part of the brain was necessary for generating sham rage, and so it's another line of evidence that supports this idea that the hypothalamus is important. And his studies also tell something about how that sham rage is controlled. What he did was he basically did experiments in which he cut the brain of an experimental animal and he cut at different places to see what parts of the brain were important for generating specific behaviors. So if you look at diagrams of how he cut the brain, what he did was he would cut in some plane and basically cut many frontal and upper regions of the brain, leaving the hypothalamus attached to the brain stem. In this situation, this is an experiment that led animals to become very sensitive to external stimuli. So for instance, if you have an animal like this and you just touch the animal, the animal, just from stroking its fur, will go into a rage and just the simple touch of that will generate rage. That's a cut in which the hypothalamus is preserved.

What Bard did in addition to this was now did another cut in another animal now cutting a little bit further back and cutting further back this time removing the hypothalamus from the rest of the nervous system. In this case the animal was placid and was not enraged, didn't react strongly to stimuli. What these two experiments show together suggest that what the hypothalamus is doing here is playing a critical, necessary role for generating rage. Furthermore the hypothalamus seems to be getting input from the part of the brain that was cut off. In other words, the hypothalamus seems to get input from the brain to control the response. In this case inhibiting the response because of course animals don't spend all their time enraged. What that means is that the hippocampus seems to be some central signaling station for receiving inputs that say it's time to be angry, it's time not to be angry, and then generating an appropriate response. That's evidence that the hypothalamus is critically involved in these very angry enraged responses.

I should say again, these are intense responses. These are far more than the simple homeostatic response. These are immediate, overwhelming responses. I've talked about emotions as being allostatic, but this is a case in which we have a negative emotion such as rage and it takes us to extremes. It's a case of, in some sense getting us back to an allostatic desired state because it's directly connected with immediate survival. These responses, rage and attack, are exceptions to the simplest idea of homeostasis. They can get us in a sense, back to normal, for instance by keeping us safe. But they can also be the end of us. All of this, including all the other responses I've talked about, are all contained in this little grape-sized gland sitting underneath the thalamus in the brain.

So that's the hypothalamus. As I've indicated from Bard's experiments, other brain regions are in the business of determining when it's time to be aggressive or even to enter a rage. So therefore it's useful to think about, well, what the other brain regions are that hold us back that start making these decisions about when it's time to be angry, when it's time to be happy, sad, and so on. Now what I'd like to do is focus on another brain region, the amygdala. We've met the amygdala before in the stress response. The amygdala, shaped like an almond therefore its name—which is the Latin word for almond—the amygdala is a region that can have a powerful suppressive effect on aggression. It seems to play a key role in driving strong emotional responses. I'll give you an example. In an animal, and also in humans, damage to the amygdala can inhibit aggression. This has been shown in animals, and in fact there are cases where this fact has been used as basically an extreme treatment of desperation in humans. People who have problems with aggression have sometimes had amygdalactomies and these amygdalactomies have been done in order to prevent aggression. Obviously that's an extreme treatment, it's in the same general category as a prefrontal lobotomy, treatments that used to be done, basically psychosurgery, to try to prevent bad behaviors. But it's now recognized that brain damage such as amygdalactomy and prefrontal lobotomy are extreme treatments that are irreversible and therefore treatments of last resort. But these treatments also tell us that the amygdala seems to play a role.

Recall that I've talked before about various ways in which the visual system is organized, and one example of what the amygdala does is organize our response to a possible dangerous stimulus. For instance, consider a hiker walking in the woods and encountering a branch, and it's a curved branch and it could be a snake. That response immediately to the branch is to jump back because it could be a snake. And that response is mediated by a rapid response from your visual system sending a signal to your amygdala saying, well you better watch out, that could be something very dangerous. So that's an example of a rapid response by the amygdala. And I've talked about the amygdala as sending signals to control the hypothalamus. The amygdala in turn also is controlled by other brain regions, and for instance, when the site of this branch is processed by other parts of your brain, you can suppress your response to this curved branch. You can say well it's not a snake, it's just a branch.

We know that the amygdala regulates responses like this and the amygdala also regulates other responses. So for instance, damage to the amygdala which I have talked about already, can reduce physical signs of anxiety. It can reduce signs of anxiety such as sweating; it can reduce responses to anxiety situations. You can tell because animals with damage to their amygdala have less vigilance, less freezing when they see something dangerous, and they're less likely to run. What this suggests is that the amygdala seems to play some important role in generating the responses associated with fear. So the amygdala plays a critical role in fear and also in generating responses such as anger.

Not everything the amygdala does is negative. The amygdala also responds rapidly to positive emotional stimuli. Say for instance you're hungry. If you're hungry and you see something edible, then your amygdala is in fact activated, and this has been seen in fMRI scans that hungry people have amygdala activity when they see something edible. After they've eaten, the amygdala is not activated by the sight of the food. So it seems like the amygdala then generates some response that's appropriate to the situation, appropriate to your state. Indeed if you look in the amygdala and you look at neurons in animals to find out what neurons respond to, neurons in the amygdala respond to various kinds of sensory information. They respond to sight, they respond to sound, and they respond to touch. Sometimes there are neurons that respond to all three. So to summarize what the amygdala seems to be doing, the amygdala seems to be important for focusing attention on emotionally salient positive or negative events in the world and directing appropriate responses. So this is a thing that the amygdala does on a moment-to-moment basis to get us through life.

In addition to generating responses, the amygdala is also important in learning, it's capable of learning. So like other parts of the nervous system that I've talked about, it is possible for the amygdala to change. In addition to generating these simple fear responses, it's also capable of learning. In fact there is a particular type of learning that involves fear conditioning and it's something that has been studied in a wide variety of animals. It is possible to teach an animal to be afraid of a neutral stimulus, and this has been seen in a wide range of animals. It has been seen in us, it has been seen in monkeys, other primates besides us, other mammals including dogs and cats and rabbits. It's been seen in birds and lizards, in fish, and even in sea slugs, Aplysia, which is a famous organism that's used for studying plasticity, and even in flies. Over and over again across animals it is possible to see conditioning of fear. You can teach an animal to be afraid of something relatively neutral, and what that suggests is that there's something deep and ancestral in learning to be afraid of something that could be dangerous. This seems to involve changes in the brain and it's likely to involve synaptic plasticity. If you look in all these animals you can see synaptic plasticity. In particular if you look in mammals, it's possible to see changes in the amygdala.

Remember I've talked before about memory. I've talked about different memory systems using different brain regions. What's suggested to be the case in fear conditioning is fear conditioning is thought to involve changes that happen in the amygdala. Therefore changes in the amygdala are important for fear conditioning. Also remember I've talked before about post-traumatic stress disorder, things that happen after a traumatic event such as rape or a terrible wartime experience. These experiences seem to be stored, at least at first, in the amygdala. It's possible to look at the amygdala and to ask the question, well let's see, how could you study this in an animal and how would you study it, for instance, in the amygdala? Here's how the experiment is typically done. The experiment is typically done with a rat standing in a cage and the cage is one in which there's a wire floor, and the animal is just walking around and then a sound comes, a relatively neutral tone. Then what happens next is that the experimenter gives a mild shock to the floor of the cage, enough for the rat to pay attention and to not like that. Rats respond to this by freezing. They stop. The next time the sound comes the animal freezes right away. In other words, this is learning that happens in one trial. One tone followed by one shock is enough to induce learning, and that's like fear learning in humans. So this kind of learning is immediate, it's not like other kinds of learning that sometimes take multiple trials, but this is a case in which one tone-shock pairing is enough to teach fear.

When the amygdala is damaged, rats and other animals lose this ability to learn fear. So what seems to be the case is that in this form of learning something changes at a cellular level. That something that changes seems to happen in the amygdala. It's possible to study this at the level of single synapses, it's possible to study this in a slice of brain tissue where you can probe connections in a brain slice and measure responses in neurons separated from the rest of the animal. It's possible to do this, for instance, by recording from one neuron in an amygdala. What neuroscientists can do is take brain tissue and keep it alive in the dish, and record from a single neuron in the amygdala, and then shock axons that bring information to the amygdala from other brain regions. For example, it's possible to shock axons from the hippocampal formation, which brings information into the amygdala, and when you shock those axons what you can do is you can measure the size of the response. Measure the size of the synaptic response and look at and measure that size of the response. What you can do is then you can give strong stimulation to that pathway, or you can pair it with activation of other pathways, and get the response size to change. This is evidence that it's possible to induce change at the level of synaptic responses in tissue by very small numbers of stimuli, sometimes a single stimulus. This is a process of synaptic plasticity, one I've talked about before. This process requires specific molecular signals at the level of biochemical changes that happen inside cells.

For example, it requires a particular type of glutamate receptor, glutamate remember being the major excitatory neurotransmitter of the brain, glutamate receptors exist on these neurons as they do on most neurons of the brain. There's a particular type of glutamate receptor called the "NMDA receptor." It's called that because it's sensitive to that particular chemical when experimenters work with it, and this particular receptor allows calcium ions to pass into cells. Those calcium ions act as a signal to drive plasticity. This is a very common motif in synaptic plasticity that some experience can be converted into a neural signal and then that's converted to a biochemical change inside cells. That biochemical change then leads to changes in the strength of the synapse by doing things like putting receptors into the membrane or by inducing other changes in the synapse. So this is a model in which it's possible to take something like fear conditioning in a rat in a cage and to start understanding steps that seem to underlie that fear conditioning at the level of single synapsis. So this is something, a case in which neuroscientists have been able to go from behavior all the way to molecular mechanisms and what individual synapses are doing.

This is how fear is learned in a single trial in this way that seems to involve changes in the amygdala. But once learned, can fear memory be unlearned? It turns out that unlearning is much harder than learning in this case. It turns out that fear conditioning is something that evolutionarily needs to be learned on a single trial because you need to know on one try. You might not get a second chance that you should watch out for that tone or the rustle of leaves that turns out to be a tiger or whatever it might be. So unlearning, however, requires many trials. It requires repeated exposure, and this other kind of learning, this unlearning, is a form of learning, and it seems to involve other structures including the hippocampus and the neocortex. An example of unlearning would be dealing with a phobia or dealing with post-traumatic stress disorder. A typical form of unlearning involves getting repeated exposure to the fear-inducing stimulus. So for instance if you're a rat the way you would do this is—you're the rat and you've heard the tone—the way that unlearning is done in a rat would be to present the tone over and over again with no bad outcome, with no shock to the feet. So that's a kind of therapy that you can do to unlearn fear.

Let's take it as an example. Let's say that you're afraid of crossing bridges. If you have a phobia of bridges, say driving across bridges, then a typical treatment would be to every day cross a bridge. It could be a bridge that you drive across, it could be a little bridge that you walk across, but every day make sure that you cross a small bridge. Eventually associating that crossing of a small bridge with no bad outcome, assuming that there's no bad outcome, will eventually help you unlearn that fear. So that's an example of repeated cognitive therapy to unlearn a fear.

There's some recent work that seems to imply that there are ways to manipulate learning mechanisms to help us unlearn a little bit more efficiently. For example, think about a fear-inducing stimulus, let's say, for instance, this bridge. If you think about a fear-inducing stimulus for 10 minutes before being presented with the prospect of actually crossing the bridge, thinking about a fear-inducing stimulus seems to enhance unlearning. This has been done in the laboratory. It's as if the learned event is effective at teaching our fear system for 10 minutes. It's as if there's some eligibility for learning that's set up by the experience of thinking about a bridge, and that there's a time window of opportunity during which unlearning can take place. What that means is that it's possible to unlearn a little bit faster by thinking about the thing that you're afraid of and then being exposed to it, and that thinking for a few minutes can enhance unlearning. Another possible treatment that researchers are interested in is to give a drug that blocks molecular mechanisms of forming long-term memories. It's possible to imagine someday that we might be able to enhance unlearning with a drug that say blocks the sensation of fear and pairing that with the innocuous stimulus.

Like other brain regions that show activity when we engage in an act and when we see someone else engage in an act, there is also a social component to how the amygdala processes fear. This is possible to see in humans who have specific damage to their amygdala. I've talked a bit about animal experiments, it turns out that it's a little bit hard to find humans with specific damage to the amygdala, but there is one case that has been documented well, and it's one that was found by Dr. Ralph Adolphs who did this work at the University of Iowa. This is the case of a 30-year-old women named SM and she had specific damage from a rare neurological disorder that led to damage to her amygdala. What she was able to do is, she had trouble identifying certain emotions in photos. This was interesting, she could easily identify people in photos, that was fine, and she was fine with identifying happiness, sadness, or disgust, and recall that I've talked about disgust in the context of the insula. But she was less good at describing an angry face and she was really bad at recognizing facial expressions of fearful faces. This is interesting because it shows that the amygdala seems to be involved not only in generating and processing these emotions in ourselves, but also in other people. So this is a recurring motif that brain regions seem to be important in processing our own emotions, our own reactions, and those of others as well.

I finally want to turn to anxiety, and anxiety of course is closely related to fear. Anxiety is expressed as a physical response that includes increased heart rate, fast breathing, and sweating. Except anxiety is in response to perceived danger as opposed to a specific event. For instance we feel anxious if we're worried about whether we left the stove on after we left the house, did we lock the door, that kind of thing. These are examples of anxiety. The amygdala is also involved in activating anxiety. It's involved in generating anxious responses. When we feel anxious, the amygdala generates a response and there's also activation of the hippocampus.

Previously I've talked about adult-acquired fear conditioning. Earlier in this lecture I talked about having a neutral stimulus generate fear conditioning in a single trial in an adult animal. This fear and anxiety system can also malfunction to cause anxiety disorders. So imagine an anxiety disorder in which you worry about everything. You worry about the plane crashing, you worry about your computer crashing, you worry about whether something bad is going to happen on the way to work. Anxiety disorders can be debilitating. They can keep people from being able to go out.

In anxiety disorders the hypothalamic pituitary adrenal axis, the same axis that we've talked about before in the context of stress, this axis shows a high level of activity. Anxiety disorders are marked by specific biochemical and neurological changes that are specific to anxiety disorder, and one major hypothesis of anxiety disorder is that this axis malfunctions. I want to link this back now to a previous lecture that I've given on personality, and remember at that time I mentioned that babies who are high reactive, fearful of things like a mobile dangled over their crib, often became anxious children or adults. Remember I said that in early life, in that first year of life, I mentioned that soothing the baby could help reduce that tendency, reduce the tendency towards fearfulness and worry. It turns out that another key period in the generation of an anxious personality, in this case in anxiety disorders, happens earlier in development before the baby is born. It has been observed that maternal stress and the secretion of stress hormones, is associated with later emotional problems, including anxiety disorders. What this suggests is that activation of stress responses, extreme stress in the mother, can affect fetal brain development to influence the likelihood of an anxiety disorder. So this is another case in which the nervous system changes in response to an event, except now we're talking about a prenatal event.

Let's summarize what we've talked about today. I've spent a lot of time talking about the hypothalamus, this Grand Central Station for allostatic responses, responses such as maintaining temperature, regulating appetite, and thirst. The hypothalamus is important in generating responses that keep us on an even keel. But it's also important and powerful in primal emotional reactions, anger and rage. Another brain region that we've spent a lot of time on is the amygdala, another key place in generating emotional responses. It's important for controlling emotional responses and it's one step upstream of the hypothalamus. The amygdala is important in handling a number of emotions including anger, also fear, and anxiety, as well as positive emotions like seeing food. In particular, I focus on fear and anxiety, things that we can either learn quickly on a very short timescale with one bad experience, or in the case of anxiety, something that can be acquired over a lifetime. In all these cases these responses, these disorders, are hard to unlearn, at least for now with current technology.

So in the next lecture what I'd like to do is take emotions down to a longer timescale and talk about the general tone of emotions that we have over long periods of time, and that's referred to as "mood."

From Weather to Climate—Mood
Lecture 28

> The weather can change from day to day, but climate takes much longer to change. Likewise, mood takes a longer time to change than emotion.

Moods are affected by environmental events: exposure to sunlight, the amount of sleep we get, our physical health. Examples of extreme moods can tell us something about the moods that we experience normally. Think of mood as a spectrum of possibilities, with mood disorders at the extreme of the spectrum. Mood, like emotion, depends on an interplay of signals between the body and the brain.

Symptoms of depression can be triggered by negative life events, such as bereavement, and by physical signals from the body, such as chronic pain. Depression as a mood disorder is recognizable by lowered mood and decreased interest or pleasure in all life activities. If these two symptoms are present every day for two weeks and no obvious life event, such as bereavement, has triggered the mood, the diagnosis is major depression.

Related to depression is bipolar syndrome, which includes depressive episodes interspersed with manic episodes that are characterized by inflated self-esteem or grandiosity, diminished need for sleep, talkativeness, racing thoughts, distractibility, and increased-goal directed activity. A milder form of mania is associated with increased efficiency, accomplishment, and creativity. Because people with bipolar syndrome often miss the manic episodes, getting them to stick with their medications can be difficult.

Several major theories and models attempt to explain what goes wrong in the brain that causes depression. One theory focuses on problems in monoamine neurotransmitters that are important in regulating mood, attention, sleep, and movement: dopamine, serotonin, adrenaline, and noradrenaline. The evidence that these molecules are involved in depression comes from drug treatments in which these neurotransmitters are manipulated pharmacologically. Blocking the breakdown of serotonin and noradrenaline with MAO inhibitors elevates mood, suggesting some role for monoamine transmitters in depression. Other pharmacological treatments include some antidepressant drugs that act directly on receptors in neurotransmitter pathways to manipulate neurotransmitter systems in the brain. One such drug influences GABA, an inhibitory neurotransmitter, by blocking GABA receptors.

Treatments that are effective for major depressive disorder include cognitive behavioral therapy, which applies specific techniques to dispel in patients negative evaluations of themselves, the world, and the future. Electroconvulsive therapy also has proven effective for major depression. It involves inducing seizures throughout the entire brain and can relieve symptoms for months. It is especially effective when paired with cognitive behavioral therapy.

Deep-brain stimulation can lead to nearly instantaneous changes in mood. The observation that depressive episodes are associated with activity in a thin strip of cortical tissue called the subgenual cingulate, or Area 25, led to a small study showing that stimulation of the **white matter** under Area 25 relieved symptoms in four out of six patients who were not helped by medication, electroconvulsive therapy, or psychotherapy.

Finally, a therapy that does not require brain surgery seems to be effective. It involves stimulation of the vagus nerve, part of the sympathetic nervous system, and helps about a third of patients who don't respond to antidepressants. The vagus nerve conveys information to the brain about body systems; thus, one hypothesis is that this treatment works because feelings of well-being may depend on the interplay between body and brain signals. This is reminiscent of the James-Lange theory that the brain sends signals to the body and the body sends physiological responses back to tell us what our mood is. ■

Important Term

white matter: Axons; in the fresh brain, the myelin sheath surrounding axons gives it a "whitish" appearance.

1. Multiple treatment options are available for depression, including cognitive behavioral therapy and antidepressants. Discuss the pros and cons of these approaches. If it were you, which would you be inclined to try first?

2. What molecule does Prozac act upon in affecting mood? How does this work, and why does it take so long?

From Weather to Climate—Mood
Lecture 28—Transcript

Welcome back. I've spent the last few lectures talking about emotion, and what I'd like to do is shift focus a little bit on the same theme, except what I'd like to do is now I'd like to turn to the theme of mood for this lecture.

We've talked about events and how they provoke emotional responses. These events can activate brain systems including amygdala, hypothalamus, and other brain regions to provoke an emotional response. In addition to those immediate responses we have emotional tone, and that emotional tone can vary on a slower timescale and can set a tone on a persistent basis, and that persistent emotional tone is mood. So one way of thinking about this is that emotion is to mood the way weather is to climate. So, the weather can change from day to day, but climate takes much longer to change. Likewise, mood takes a longer time to change than emotion. So if we think about our daily moodiness, we have good moods, we have bad moods. Perhaps if we're hungry we're in a bad mood so that would be an example of the brain's hunger system affecting our mood. If you haven't had your caffeine if you're a coffee drinker, maybe you're in a bad mood before you've had your morning coffee. Moods are then affected by environmental events. They're affected by exposure to sunlight, they're affected by the amount of sleep we get, our physical health. To give an example, for instance one mood disorder, depression is very common in people with chronic pain. So nearly everybody with chronic pain is depressed.

For purposes of this course, what I'd like to do is shed light on everyday moods, our normal mood changes by exploring what happens when we get to the extremes of mood. What we'll do in this coming lecture is talk about moods at the extremes, and so I've mentioned depression, but also giddy mania and swings between the two, bipolar disorder. These are examples of extreme moods that can tell us something about the moods that we normally experience. I want you to think of mood as a spectrum of possibilities. A mood disorder then would be something that's at the extreme of the spectrum, something where we would not normally want to spend all our time. So our moods are this emotional tone that moves along the spectrum. Now that's a contrast of something like schizophrenia, or dementia such as Alzheimer's disease, where a function is very clearly outside the range of normal function and is in a place where we basically don't explore in daily life.

Some moods are not really considered dysfunctional, so it's possible to classify a mood in some clinical sense and yet it's not dysfunctional. In fact, some of these moods can be considered positively functional. For example, I'll be talking about something called "hypomania." This is a mood in which people need less sleep, are very talkative, and are very goal directed. In modern life, hypomania is often not considered to be a bad thing. Now let's discuss mood disorders. Mood disorders first become apparent at puberty. I've mentioned this before when talking about childhood and adolescence, there's something about the brain maturation process that seems to make teenagers vulnerable for the first time to a wide variety of psychiatric disorders. With adolescents, there's a gradual increase in the risk of mood disorders and psychosis. For example, rates of depression and anxiety disorders begin to increase around puberty and reach adult levels by age 18. Similarly other disorders such as schizophrenia, people who are diagnosed with schizophrenia in their 20s often turn out to have exhibited their initial symptoms during adolescence. Adolescence is also a time when gender differences in these disorders start to emerge. There seems to be a role for sex hormones such as estrogen and testosterone in driving brain changes that make a disorder more or less likely. For example, mood disorders are twice as likely to occur in women than in men. Again this is something that begins around puberty. So there's something about puberty that increases the risk of brain dysfunction in many ways, and in particular mood disorders. It's not really all that well understood, at least not yet.

Mood, like emotion, is dependent on an interplay of signals between the body and the brain. So we've talked about the James Lange affair, we've talked about the Cannon-Bard theory in which the brain and body talk to one another to generate emotions. Mood is the same story except in the case of mood that conversation can take place on longer timescales. For example, symptoms of depression can be triggered by negative life events such as bereavement or some other intense bad event. Depression can also be triggered by physical signals from the body, as I've mentioned chronic pain. So therefore we should think of mood as being critically dependent on not only the brain, but also on signals that come from the body.

These mood disorders are, in fact, fairly common in the general population. Estimates of mood disorders in the general population include the likelihood of having a major depressive episode in any given year is about 7 percent. The lifetime risk of having a mood disorder sometime in your lifetime is between 1 in 10 to as high as 2 in 10, so a 10 to 20 percent risk of a major mood disorder, a major depressive episode, in your lifetime. That's a fairly considerable risk.

Let's talk about depression then, because it's something that's likely to happen either to you or perhaps to somebody who you care about. Depression is not just feeling down. It's not just a transient problem. It's an actual medical disorder and it's recognizable as a medical disorder by the following symptoms. The main symptoms of depression are lowered mood and decreased interest or pleasure in all life activities. A diagnosis of major depression comes if these two symptoms are present every day for two weeks and there's no obvious life event such as bereavement to have triggered the mood, because of course it would be a natural response to something like bereavement. There are other symptoms that come with major depression and one can go through them and so let's think about them. The other symptoms of major depression include loss of appetite, or perhaps increased appetite; insomnia or hypersomnia; sleeping too little or sleeping too much; fatigue; feelings of worthlessness or guilt; a diminished ability to concentrate; recurrent thoughts of death for instance suicide and of course obviously a suicide attempt. Also persistent aches or pains, headaches, cramps or digestive problems, things that are unpleasant and do not ease even with treatment. All of these are signs of depression, and if five or more of these signs appear and persisted for several weeks, then that would be again an indicator of depression.

Depression plays out in different ways. Different people react to depression in different ways. For instance, despair would be one reaction to depression and that's more common in women. Another example of a response to depression would be aggression or self-destructive behavior, and that's more common in men. Depression is quite common in the population, as I've said, and it also is exceptionally common in very accomplished people. For instance, accomplished artists show a very high rate of major depression many times higher than the general public. You can find it in other prominent figures as well. For instance, Winston Churchill went through episodes of depression and he called it his "black dog." The writer F. Scott Fitzgerald found himself, "hating the night when I couldn't sleep and hating the day because it went toward night." These are experiences that are felt by many people and as I said you can see it, for instance, in biographical studies of accomplished artists.

Related to depression is something similar which is bipolar syndrome. Bipolar syndrome is something that's less common, it only affects less than 2 percent of the population. Bipolar syndrome includes depressive episodes and these depressive episodes are as I've described them before. But in addition to depressive episodes, mood can move up or down and this up/down movement of mood can take place over a period of weeks or months. The up phases are very different from depression. The up phase is known as "mania," and manic episodes include the following signs: inflated self-esteem or grandiosity; diminished need for sleep; talkativeness or perhaps an impulsive need to talk and fill silences; flight of ideas or racing thoughts; and finally distractibility. In addition to these, also increased goal directed activity. In fact, one version of mania is hypomania, so a milder form of mania. This is a minority of people with bipolar syndrome, people who are hypomanic. In this case the symptoms I just talked about, which honestly sound kind of fun—talkativeness, increased activity—they can be associated in the milder form with increased efficiency, accomplishment, and creativity. So often it's the case that people with hypomania in fact like the fact that they have up and down swings.

Let's take as an example the composer Robert Schumann. During his lifetime Robert Schumann had wildly fluctuating outputs. So in some years he wrote many, many compositions, and in other years not. So for instance, he had a hypomanic episode in 1849 and in that year that was the most productive year of his career, he wrote 27 compositions. Compare that with 1844, five years earlier, this is a year in which he had no compositions. So during his career he went between wild extremes in his output. That's an example of hypomania.

Another example of hypomania is the writer Virginia Woolf. Her husband describes how, "she talked almost without stopping for two or three days, paying no attention to anyone in the room or anything said to her." So these are extreme experiences that can often lead to not only great function, but in fact, dysfunction. They sometimes are described as these momentary bright spots in what is otherwise a very unpleasant experience because depression, after all, is horrible. So for instance, Robert Lowell said that manic experiences were, for him, like, "a magical orange grove in a nightmare." So his landscape of depression was punctuated by these events that were just wonderful for him. It's often the case that, in fact, people who are treated for bipolar syndrome don't necessarily like being treated because they miss the hypomanic or manic episodes. They like the manic episodes and they miss them. So one thing that's seen in the medical treatment of bipolar syndrome is that it's often hard to get bipolar people to stick with their meds because they miss the hypomanic episodes.

It's important to note that bipolar syndrome is very different from depression. The causes are not well understood, but what's important is that reactions to medication are different in bipolar syndrome compared with depression. For instance if you give Prozac, a common antidepressant, to a bipolar syndrome, it is possible that that person could become suicidal. It's not clear why that is. A better treatment is lithium, this salt that is related to sodium, and lithium gets into cells and interferes with second messenger signaling. So it interferes with all the signals that come as a downstream consequence of metabotropic receptor activation, neurotransmitters such as serotonin, dopamine, noradrenaline. This process seems to be interfered with by lithium, and that seems to be helpful in the case of treating bipolar syndrome.

Now let's go back to depression, let's talk about depression and what may cause depression. There are several major theories and models for what goes wrong in the brain that causes depression, what takes us to this extreme of mood? One category of phenomena that seem to be involved in depression is problems in monoamine neurotransmitters. I've named a few of them just now. These monoamine neurotransmitters are important in regulating mood, but also attention, sleep, and movement. I've mentioned these monoamines several times in this series of lectures in this course, and they include dopamine, serotonin, adrenaline, and noradrenaline. These molecules have lots of jobs despite the fact that they are made by only a tiny fraction of the neurons of the brain. They seem to be involved in anxiety; mood;

schizophrenia; stress, as we've heard several times; Huntington's disease; Parkinson's; sleep disorders. They are busy, busy molecules.

The evidence that these molecules are involved in depression comes from drug treatments in which these neurotransmitters, these monoamines, are manipulated pharmacologically. Some of the earliest evidences comes from a drug that's an old blood pressure medication called "reserpine." Serotonin gets its original name because it was found to alter blood vessel tone, serotonin. Depleting serotonin with reserpine, which is this old blood pressure medication, was observed to cause psychotic depression in 20 percent of patients. So a major side effect leading to less use of reserpine and the advent of other blood pressure medications.

Conversely, blocking the breakdown of several of these molecules, specifically serotonin and noradrenaline, can be done by giving a drug that blocks the enzyme monoamine oxidase. This is an enzyme whose job it is to break down monoamines. "MAO" is a name that you may encounter when you read about drugs. Blocking the breakdown of these neurotransmitters with MAO inhibitors elevates mood. These pieces of evidence suggest that there is some role for monoamine transmitters in determining mood, and specifically they may go out of range in the phenomenon of depression.

Another possible brain system that seems to be involved in depression is alterations in the stress response. We've spent a fair amount of time talking about the stress response, the stress response recall, being important in homeostatic adaptation and also things like getting away from danger. Mood disorders run in families and our genes can predispose us to mental illness, including depression. But also there's another familial role in generating a mood disorder and we've talked about it before, which is early childhood neglect or life stresses, early childhood abuse, and including maternal stress prenatally. These events are big risk factors in the development of mood disorders. In particular, high activity in the hypothalamic pituitary adrenal system is often seen in anxiety disorders as I mentioned before in a previous lecture, and high activity in the HPA system is also seen in depression.

It turns out that there are a number of effective treatments for depression, and some of these are based on these models for depression that I've just described. Each of them can be effective even when the other treatments fail. So even if one treatment for depression fails, it's possible to try another treatment. It seems to be the case that success of one treatment is not dependent on whether another one has succeeded or failed, and so it's necessary when dealing with depression to think about all the possible treatments.

First let's talk about mild depressive symptoms. This is something that's more likely to happen in everyday life. There are things that we can do in everyday life to alter our mood, to raise or to lower it, and these are important to think about just for improving the quality of our everyday lives. Recall when I talked about aging and I talked about the physical benefits of physical exercise on brain fitness. Exercise is also associated with reduced anxiety and reduced likelihood of depression, including in young adults and adolescents. So exercise is a thing that can be done for dealing with mild depressive symptoms. Another thing that can be done to deal with mild depressive symptoms is sleep. Disrupted sleep is a risk factor for mild depression, and therefore sleep is something that one can engage in to reduce the risk of depression.

Just as an aside I want to mention that there is some funny business with sleep. There is some literature suggesting the converse, and this is an interesting phenomenon. In cases of severe depression there is a treatment that seems to work immediately to reduce the symptoms of severe depression and it's sleep deprivation. This is very strange, and so there seems to be some very short-term effect of sleep to reduce the symptoms of depression. It seems to work in part by inhibition of the anterior cingulate cortex. So we've talked about the anterior cingulate before in the interpretation of pain and of emotions and inhibition of emotional responses. What's seen in brain scans is that sleep deprivation leads to decreased activity in the anterior cingulate cortex. It seems as if acute sleep deprivation, just staying up all night, seems to remove that inhibition. It's like taking a foot off the brake, and it's as if inhibition is removed and then that disinhibition improves the mood. The unfortunate part of this particular treatment is that the moment you take a nap the depression returns. It's sort of like putting on a tourniquet to stop bleeding, it's okay, but only as an emergency short-term treatment.

Now let's go back to mild depression. Other treatments for mild depressive episodes include having regular habits including not only sleep, but also rising early. The reason for rising early is that sunlight seems to play a role in affecting mood. There's a phenomenon known as "seasonal affective disorder," and this is more commonly found in upper latitudes, for instance in Scandinavian countries where days get very short in winter. Those short days seem to be associated with increased incidents of depression in wintertime. For instance, people in Finland are more prone to depression and less happy, on average, than people in Denmark. All of these treatments can also help with anxiety. Recall that I've talked about anxiety, and a lot of the neuromechanisms of depression are overlapping with those for anxiety.

Now let's turn to major depressive disorder. This is the kind of depression that I talked about before where people have depressed mood for two weeks, general lack of enjoyment of everyday life. There are treatments that are effective for the treatment of major depressive disorder. The most effective of these is something that doesn't involve any drugs at all, and it's known as "cognitive behavioral therapy," "CBT." It turns out that CBT is effective and works well for about one-third of depressed persons, and so CBT is the first choice for dealing with a major depressive episode.

Much cognitive behavioral therapy is based on the idea that depressed individuals make negative evaluations of themselves, the world, and the future. This negative evaluation leads to a negative interpretation of events. So the general idea in cognitive behavioral therapy is to apply specific techniques to get individuals away from that kind of thinking, and this can take multiple forms. For instance, one activity in CBT is to keep a diary of significant events and feelings and to question thoughts and assumptions and interpretations that are unhelpful or unrealistic. To review one's thoughts and reevaluate how one reacts to events. Another part of CBT is to face activities that were being avoided, and so if you're avoiding an activity, just face up to it and get in there and go do it. Other techniques include trying out new ways of behaving and reacting to events. Finally, relaxation, mindfulness, and distraction techniques, ways to get you off the negative thoughts, ways to get you away from whatever negative feelings that you have.

It turns out that one thing that's interesting about CBT is that the therapy is effective both for mild and severe depression. Not only is it effective for depressive episodes, but it can even be applied to day-to-day moods and so it's possible to apply the techniques of cognitive behavioral therapy to day-to-day moods just as you can apply it to clinical conditions. In fact, one can find examples of this in spiritual teachings. One can look at the Buddha as an early cognitive therapist because he was interested in helping ordinary people deal with ordinary everyday life.

Another category of treatment, finally, is pharmacological, and this gets back to what I was talking about with the monoamine hypothesis of depression and of other mood disorders. There are antidepressant drugs that act directly by acting on receptors in neurotransmitter pathways to manipulate neurotransmitter systems in the brain. There are many types of these. So for instance, one category is drugs that deal with GABA receptors and so these are receptors that are inhibitory, GABA is an inhibitory neurotransmitter. There are antidepressants that specifically act on GABA receptors as if what's being done is removing inhibition in the brain, again, taking a foot off the brake. Other categories of antidepressant drugs include drugs that deal with monoamine neurotransmitters, so drugs that interfere with or deal with norepinephrine, dopamine, and serotonin. One major category is serotonin uptake inhibitors, these drugs like Prozac, Paxil, and other drugs that specifically block the vacuuming up of serotonin after it has been released. So the site of action of these drugs is that Prozac acts upon some transporter for serotonin and prevents serotonin from being vacuumed back up. That's a way of dealing with depression.

There's something odd about this, which is that Prozac's action takes weeks. It requires repeated use over many weeks to take effect. That's a little bit odd, and what it suggests is that there's something a little bit mysterious, something that we don't really quite understand, about how Prozac affects mood. What seems to be the case is that brain neurochemistry adapts to the repeated administration of these drugs and it somehow seems to be the case that there's some compensatory mechanism that the brain has for dealing with all that extra serotonin. One proof of this is that there's another drug that blocks serotonin uptake, but it is not used for this purpose and doesn't do the same thing, and it's a drug called "MDMA," also known as "ecstasy."

Ecstasy is used in clubs and it's a drug that's specifically used to generate feelings of ecstasy and of love towards other people. Surprisingly, MDMA has the same effect on the same molecular target, and the reason this is surprising is that ecstasy's effects are short lived. They're typically less than 12 hours and ecstasy also blocks the action of the serotonin transporter. So why is it that Prozac and ecstasy have such different effects? Why is it that a single dose of Prozac does not lead to ecstasy-like effects? One possibility is that despite the fact that they have the same molecular targets, they enter the brain at different rates. So for instance, if Prozac gets to the brain more slowly than ecstasy, it might not give the same initial rush. Ecstasy also turns out to block other receptors, it turns out to block dopamine uptake. So there's a possibility that in fact these drugs have somewhat different modes of activity in the brain.

I now want to turn to some extreme therapies that seem to be surprisingly effective in dealing with depression. One kind of therapy that has worked surprisingly well for depression is electroconvulsive therapy, shock therapy. This is a very effective therapy for major depression and it basically involves inducing seizures throughout the entire brain. Inducing these seizures can relieve symptoms for months and it's especially effective when paired with cognitive behavioral therapy. This is interesting because it's a fairly extreme treatment for depression and is currently given by giving people sedations so that they don't hurt themselves, and then inducing seizures in the brain. Then afterwards people report fairly significant elevation of mood and the lifting of the darkness. It's not known why this works because it's something that is basically a seizure throughout the entire brain.

More recently there have been more specific treatments that are more focused, more refined, that seem to also have an effect on depression. I'm quite excited about this because some of these involve getting into specific brain regions that might be very directly involved in the generation of mood and depression. For instance there's one category of treatment called "deep brain stimulation." Deep brain stimulation can lead to near instantaneous changes in mood such as depression or mania. Deep brain stimulation is a treatment that's used to treat disorders such as Parkinson's disease. A surgeon can go into the brain, into the subthalamic nucleus, to look for a region that can help with Parkinson's disease. But there's a case in which a surgeon missed by 2 mm, by one-tenth of an inch, and the surgeon hit a region that led to intense mania. Another case was one in which stimulation led to intense depression, weeping and saying things like, "I'm disgusted with life, everything is useless, always feeling worthless, I'm scared in this world." This is awful, just the idea of inducing depression. But in that case the patient's symptoms disappeared and she felt much better a minute after the stimulation ended.

Another case is the activation of basically hypomania. Again just a few millimeters away missing the desired target, the result is something along the lines of mania. In this case this patient reported euphoria, non-stop talking, grandiose delusions, increased sexual drive. In this case the positive effects, the manic effects, lasted for days. One of these patients asked repeatedly, well why didn't you do this procedure to me earlier? I should say at this point that this operation is not available as an elective procedure so don't go asking your doctor for this.

One thing that is unavoidable from examining case studies like these, these deep brain stimulation studies, is that it's becoming increasingly clear that we don't know much about what these deep brain regions do, these regions of the midbrain and the brain stem. These brain regions are incredibly crowded places. When you look at pictures of the neocortex you can see this nice sheet that's folded up, but when you get down to the brain stem, these are regions that are closely packed with one another, little nuclei piles of cells that are next to each other. They're basically cheek-by-jowl, and there' something about it, it's like a crowded old phone switchboard and it's all this stuff packed in there. So scientifically speaking one can look at these cases of induced mania and depression as lucky accidents since these surgeons' fortuitous discoveries in the middle of the brain would never be permitted as planned research. But these brain regions are jam packed places, and when it comes down it, we don't have any real idea of what a lot of these regions do. So these accidental treatments are major opportunities, and there's a big challenge here about finding out what these brain regions do.

Here's another version of deep brain stimulation, and now this is one that was done a little bit more by design as opposed to being found by accident. This is now in the neocortex which, as I said, is a place where regions are farther apart and it's possible to poke around without accidentally missing as often. One form of deep brain stimulation therapy has been developed for the neocortex, and it's based on the observation that depressive episodes are associated with activity in a thin strip of cortical tissue called the "subgenual cingulate." This is in the anterior part of the cingulate cortex, so again anterior cingulate, and the genu is part of the corpus callosum at the midline. Underneath the genu is the subgenual cingulate.

So this is an area also known as "Area 25." Area 25 is another technical name for this area, and it becomes less active in patients who suffer from depression who don't respond to antidepressant drugs. There has been a small study in which deep brain stimulation of the white matter under Area 25, so if you go in with a probe and go there, it's possible to relieve symptoms in four out of six patients with depression who were not helped by medication, who were not helped by electroconvulsive therapy, or by psychotherapy. It's another example of direct activation of brain tissue.

Finally another version of nerve stimulation. I've talked before about the body and the brain talking with one another and sending messages back and forth as part of emotional response. There's a therapy that's less extreme than these other therapies that does not involve brain surgery and going into the brain. It seems to be effective, but it also is rather mysterious and it involves stimulation of the vagus nerve. The vagus nerve is part of the sympathetic nervous system. Vagus nerve stimulation helps about one-third of persons suffering from depression, again, a third of people who don't respond to antidepressant drugs. This is interesting because it is noninvasive to the brain, and furthermore for a time it was approved by at least one insurance company. It's sufficiently well tested in the literature that an insurance company felt that there was enough evidence in the literature to go for vagal nerve stimulation.

Why does it work? Well, evidently it involves some kind of brain-body interaction, but exactly why it works is not all that well understood. The vagus nerve conveys information to the brain about body systems, and it conveys information such as how fast the heart is beating, pain signals, information from the gut and stomach, for instance information about whether the stomach is full. So one hypothesis is that this treatment works because feelings of wellbeing may depend on the interplay between body and brain signals. In other words, vagus nerve stimulation might send happy body signals to the brain, and this is reminiscent of the James Lange theory that we talked about several lectures ago in which the brain sends signals to the body and the body sends signals, physiological responses back, to tell us what our mood is. So perhaps there's a way to understand vagus nerve stimulation in terms of old theories of emotion.

So let's summarize what we've talked about today. Mood we've talked about, and mood is something that varies on slower timescales than emotions. Mood varies over the course of a day. There's a range of emotions, but when mood gets to an extreme, dysfunctions of mood constitute major psychiatric problems. Mood is connected with, of course, emotional brain mechanisms. In particular there seems to be a connection with serotonin- based signaling mechanisms. Finally I've talked about treatments for depression and other mood disorders, treatments in which one can manipulate the mood system by drugs, by surgery. What appears to be the case is that in some cases there's evidence that the brain talks to the body, but the body talks back, and also there's evidence that there are environmental influences on our moods.

In the next lecture what I'd like to do is move on and talk about social phenomena and social thinking by our brains, the social brain.

The Social Brain, Empathy, and Autism
Lecture 29

In our species, a major part of our identity depends on the fact that we're social animals, that we have this ability to imagine the thoughts of others. ... [This] ability to model other person's mental states and what other people might be thinking, this ability is necessary for us to navigate everyday life.

Theory of mind is observed in most children by age 3 or 4. It's possible to ask a 3-year-old, or even a younger child, why he or she was crying and receive a plausible answer. How does the theory of mind develop? A possible answer to this question lies in a developmental disorder in which the capacity for theory of mind seems to be absent: autism. Autism presents several classic signs: lack of social reciprocity, disrupted verbal and nonverbal communication, and inflexible and repetitive behaviors.

Autism is mostly a genetic disorder. The exact details of the genetic inheritance suggest that more than one gene is involved in autism, and many of these genes encode brain functions: perhaps proteins found in synapses or electrical signaling in neurons or in the development of the nervous system. One current area of challenge and research is to understand how these genetic variations combine to lead to autism.

Autistic people often show perceptual deficits, such as an inappropriate degree of sensitivity to routine sounds and even to the feel of their own clothing. The perceptual deficits by themselves are less germane than the possibility that they have a deeper meaning. Recent studies have shown that perceptual problems show up very early, even in 2-year-olds, and that these children show possible perceptual problems with biological motion. This is important because biological motion is a means by which we identify persons in our environment, as opposed to inanimate objects.

Perceptual problems in autistic children also appear in other aspects of life. For example, an autistic child listening to an adult tends to look at the adult's mouth rather than the eyes. This phenomenon suggests that perceptual problems may prevent autistic children from getting social cues in the first place. In fact, one possibility is that the perceptual problems might be a root cause of the difficulty babies and children have in forming social models. Other possibilities are that perceptual dysfunction and empathetic social deficits may share some common developmental issue important in generating both of these capacities.

One brain region where deficits are visible is the amygdala, which is important in processing emotional states of others and in generating emotional responses.

One brain region where deficits are visible is the amygdala, which is important in processing emotional states of others and in generating emotional responses. Another is the **cerebellum**, a brain structure that regulates movement and seems to be involved in detecting unexpected events. There has also been speculation about the insular cortex and mirror neurons, but evidence about the involvement of these brain regions is lacking.

One of the central challenges in neuroscience research in general is to understand different levels of function, understanding how molecules work together to generate functional synapses, how neurons talk with one another, how systems of circuits work together, and how the whole works together to make a working brain. Another area of current research is the study of how developmental processes coordinate these brain regions to work separately and together over development and throughout life to generate our many capacities and the ability to think about the motivations of other people. Autism is an active area of research both for its medical importance and at a fundamental level in understanding how these processes develop and how they can go wrong. ■

Important Terms

cerebellum: Part of the metencephalon; involved in motor coordination and some cognitive functions.

theory of mind: The understanding that other individuals have different thoughts and knowledge than you; most frequently used as a term in child development.

Questions to Consider

1. What is theory of mind? Why would the amygdala be involved in this capacity?

2. What traits do autism and Asperger's syndrome share? What is known about the causes of these disorders?

The Social Brain, Empathy, and Autism
Lecture 29—Transcript

Welcome back. Over the course of the last lectures we've considered different brain systems and we've gotten into the territory of talking about some fairly complex phenomena. Phenomena that impinge on our everyday lives in ways that we're quite aware of, and we've talked about personality, intelligence, emotions, and mood. Now what I'd like to do is consider an ability that's highly remarkable, one that's highly developed in us, and one that is found in very few other species. Yet, it's quite possible that you may not have even considered it as being a separate function of the brain, a function generated by your brain. This ability that I'm talking about is the ability to imagine another person's thoughts and motivations, the ability for me to have a mental model of another person, you for instance. That ability is often referred to as "theory of mind."

What I'd like to do is to talk about this ability in the context of a disorder in which the ability is absent, and that disorder is autism. That's really notable because it's really in the absence of this capacity that we really notice how important and how essential it is for our everyday lives. What I'd like to do is focus on theory of mind through the lens of examining autism. I'll talk about how brain systems may be dysfunctional, specific brain systems that may underlie the theory of mind, may be dysfunctional in this inherited disorder. I'd like to illuminate the principle of theory of mind by comparison to how a non-autistic brain generates this remarkable ability to imagine another person's mind, so I'd like you to think of autism as a way of understanding your own mind.

In our species, a major part of our identity depends on the fact that we're social animals, that we have this ability to imagine the thoughts of others. For example, you're exercising your theory of mind perhaps as you watch this, definitely as you watch this. As you watch or listen to this lecture you might have thoughts about what I might be thinking right now. Certainly I have a mental model of people watching this lecture. I have a mental model of things that you might be thinking about, and this ability to form models about other people's mental states is called "theory of mind," that ability to model other person's mental states and what other people might be thinking.

This ability is necessary for us to navigate everyday life. For instance, it plays a critical role in the ability to empathize with others. It's critical for engaging in social and even moral reasoning. It's worthwhile, as I've done in several other lectures, to think about what non-human animals seem to have this theory of mind. Let's consider close relatives to our species, chimpanzees and orangutans.

Like us, chimpanzees are highly social animals. Chimpanzees are constantly having to guess what other chimps are thinking. For example, when a low-ranking chimp has a choice between two pieces of fruit, and a dominant chimp can only see one of them because of a barrier, then the low-ranking chimp will go for the one that the dominant chimp cannot see. What that suggests is that the low-ranking chimp has some idea of what the dominant chimp can see. Chimps are constantly engaging in complex social interactions and so in fact they engage in fairly complex reasoning including things like forming alliance with one another, ganging up on one another, saying, well I'm your friend but I'm only your friend when this other one is not present, but when they're present then I will be two-faced. So chimps engage in fairly complex social modeling and that's an example of theory of mind.

Now there's some evidence that dogs may have theory of mind as well, and I want to tell you as story about a friend's dog. The dog's name was Osa. At one point in Osa's life she was injured and she needed to be carried up and down stairs in this apartment that my friend Chris lived in. When it was time to go up or down stairs she would wait at the stairs and wait for him to pick her up and then carry her up or down stairs. This went on for weeks after she recuperated from this injury. One day Chris was puttering around quietly in the kitchen, he was just cutting something or cooking something, and he was just in the kitchen and Osa came down the stairs, perfectly able-bodied. She came down the stairs, turned the corner and saw Chris, and said—well, she didn't say anything, but she paused and she had a look that said I'm caught. That look generated in Chris the feeling that Osa had a model for whether Chris thought that it was necessary to carry her down the stairs. So that episode demonstrates the possibility of dogs have theory of mind.

I should say that there is more than just anecdotal evidence. I've just given you this story to illustrate how you might see capacity for theory of mind in another animal. But there are, in fact, studies that seem to demonstrate that dogs have some capacity for theory of mind.

It's not known how the brain generates this capacity. The mechanisms for this are not understood, except of course for the fact that the brain does generate theory of mind. So what would be a step in understanding how the brain generates theory of mind? Well, one first step might be to find brain activity that corresponds to mental states in which we have to imagine what other people are doing. What I'd like to do is review some of that evidence for you.

There are brain regions that I have, in fact, mentioned in previous lectures that are important in generating models of what other people are doing or that seem like they would be well suited for that. For instance in recent lectures I've mentioned brain regions such as the insular cortex, the insula, and also the amygdala. These brain regions are active in processing one's own emotional state, for instance, the feeling of fear or anxiety or anger. They're also important in detecting those same emotional states in other people, for instance using facial expressions, for instance, the insula for recognizing a disgusted face or the amygdala in recognizing an afraid or angry face. So those are brain regions that seem to meet the criterion of processing the mental states of other people.

Another example is something that has been in the news quite a lot in neuroscience news stories, and that's mirror neurons. Mirror neurons are interesting because they recognize actions. They recognize actions carried out by ourselves and also carried out by others. So for instance if I were to pick up a cup and drink from it, there might be neurons in my brain that are activated in correlation with that, and when I see someone else drinking from a cup, those same neurons might be activated. These mirror neurons have been seen in monkeys. They've been seen in premotor cortex, so this part of the cortex that's in front of the motor cortex, and also in another part of the neocortex, the inferior parietal cortex. So there's clear evidence from mirror neurons in monkeys, and there's some evidence in humans from scanning data that there's evidence for mirror-like activity in different parts of the brain. So mirror neurons are interesting because again they seem to encode the idea of dual function, so this idea that there are dual function neurons that seem to encode the concept of an action whether we do it or whether other people do it. These might be important for learning about actions of others, and in the case of these emotional regions, the insula and the amygdala, may be motives too. So these are just two examples that are already known from neurophysiology and from others from neuroanatomical data, There may be more in addition to these, but these are the ones that are currently known about and that are objects of active research.

Theory of mind is observed in most children by age three or four. It's possible to ask a three-year-old or even earlier, about motivations. You can say well, why did that child cry? Well, she cried because she was hurt. So it's possible to quiz children about theory of mind and get a report that they seem to have some capacity for theory of mind at that age. Of course recall that I've talked about early development in which it's now known that one can probe for these things earlier in life, and so it's possible that it exists earlier, but certainly by the age of three or four it exists.

How does the theory of mind develop? Well, as I've said at the beginning, a possible answer to this question can be seen in a developmental disorder in which the capacity for theory of mind seems to be absent and that's, as I said, autism. The ways in which brains go off track from typical paths of development in autism perhaps can tell us a lot about who we are. Autism was not discovered all that long ago. It was discovered in 1943 and named by Leo Kanner. Leo Kanner noticed that there were several classic signs of autism. He discovered the following three classic signs. The first sign was a lack of social reciprocity. The second sign was disrupted verbal and nonverbal communication. The third sign was inflexible and repetitive behaviors, things like, for instance self-stimulation where children will just do the same thing over and over again, so repetitive behaviors.

Before the discovery of autism, the language disability led to a categorization of autism as being something else, as being delayed language development. True autism, of the type that's debilitating, occurs at an incidence of about one or two kids out of a thousand. This diagnosis rate has been one or two out of a thousand, but it turns out that rates of autism and autism-related disorders has gone up in the population in the last few decades. One possible reason is that there are therapies that have been found that can help a little bit, behavioral therapies in which children can learn at an early age to perform better at some of these social interactive tasks. The existence of those therapies may perhaps motivate parents of unusually behaving children to seek a diagnosis.

So now today there are problems in addition to autism, which as I said is about one or two out of a thousand, but there are other problems that resemble autism in some ways. For instance, a major example is Asperger's disease. Persons with Asperger's syndrome have language function and are often of average intelligence or even higher, but they often have obsessions. Broadly speaking there are other kinds of disorders. For instance there's one pervasive developmental disorder not otherwise specified, this mouthful of a syndrome that you can find in handbooks of psychiatric problems. Very broadly these problems are together called "autism spectrum disorder." Today the diagnosed rate of autism spectrum disorder has been quite high, 1 in 150, and in some places even as high as 1 in 100.

Autism spectrum disorder then has become of increasing interest and it has attracted a lot of attention in various years. Therefore you've likely heard a lot about autism and its possible causes in news reports. Over the years there have been different ideas for what leads to autism. You can find theories littering the history of autism even since 1943 about what causes autism. For instance, one example is an old theory called "the refrigerator mother hypothesis." The idea is that a cold unloving mother can lead to autism, somehow the idea that having a mean mom can lead to autism. Now it's known that that's not true. What's known now to be true is autism is mostly a genetic disorder. In other words, as I said when talking about early development, development in children's brains happens largely normally with the exception of some deficit, some genetic defect that arises basically at fertilization.

What's the evidence that autism is mostly genetic? Well, the way that we tease apart whether autism has a genetic component is like what I've talked about before in the case of personality and intelligence. The way to look at it, the way to test for it, is to look at identical twins. What has been found in identical twins is that if one twin has autistic spectrum disorder, then the other is highly likely to also have autistic spectrum disorder. The likelihood of coincidence of autism in identical twins is between 50 and as high as 90 percent. So there is a high, high coincidence of autism spectrum between identical twins. This is not true of non-identical twins. For instance, if you have a pair of nonidentical twins the likelihood of an autistic nonidentical having a twin who's also autistic spectrum is higher than the general population, but much less than 50 percent. So non-identical twins who share half as much genetic information with one another are only moderately likely to both be autistic.

When scientists have looked at the exact details of the numbers of this, the exact numbers underlying identicals and non-identicals, and siblings for that matter, the exact details of the genetic inheritance suggests that there's more than one gene involved in autism. They suggest that autism can be caused in any given person by 2 to, say, as many as 10 genes. So it's better to think about it from a genetic standpoint as being kind of like an inverse lottery. The idea is that if you draw genes out of a hat and you get some from mom, some from dad, if you get the wrong combination, then in fact you're at risk for autism.

Some of these genes have been found through genetic analysis of families with autistic persons, and this is a very active area of research. What's known so far is that many of these genes encode brain functions. For instance, many of these genes encode proteins that are found in synapses. Or perhaps they encode proteins that are involved in electrical signaling in neurons such as these ion channels that I talked about very early in this course. Finally there are proteins that are involved in the development of the nervous system. So there are many of these proteins and one current area of challenge and research on autism is to understand how these genetic variations combine in just certain combinations to lead to autism.

That part is an area of active research, what's not known is how it happens. But what is known is when these combinations, these bad combinations, start having a noticeable effect on behavior. It turns out that these signs emerge early, as early as one year of age. One source of information is to look at first-year birthday party videos of children reacting at first birthday parties. Many families have first birthday party videos. Another thing you can do is to start doing behavioral tests with children and to start doing things like playing peek-a-boo with them. For instance one example of what you can do with a one-year-old is notice that he or she—autistic kids are typically male—but look at what he or she does in response to a simple game like peek-a-boo. This is something that's quite striking. If you take a child and say peek-a-boo, peek-a-boo—when you play peek-a-boo with the children, most children, typical children, will look at the person's face. But an autistic child will look at the obstacle, because that's the thing that's changing. That change seems to be the thing that's interesting to an autistic person. So that's one thing that arises quite early in autistic persons. In fact, it has been found that it's possible to identify individual babies as early as four months of age who show behavioral differences that identify them as potentially being at high-risk of autism and then to follow up. The follow up has shown that many of these children have autism.

What's striking in autistic persons in general is that there's this imagining of other's capacity that's absent. So I've given you an example of peek-a-boo where the child is as interested in the obstacle as in the face. The general capacity that seems to be absent in autistic persons is that particular imagining of others' capacity. Other functions seem close to normal. For instance, autistic persons seem to have basic sensation, they have the ability to make plans, they have the ability to act upon the plans. So a lot of capacities are still there. It's really striking that there's a social deficit and a theory of mind deficit in autistic persons.

In recent years it has been appreciated that there's another thing that's different in autistic persons, and that other thing that's different is perceptual abilities. It has now been possible to identify perceptual deficits in autism, again going back to a fairly early age. It's possible to look at toddlers and others, basically at the age of two, to find perceptual deficits in autism.

Here's the general perceptual deficit, the observation is as follows. Autistic people often show perceptual deficits such as an inappropriate degree of sensitivity to routine sounds, and even to the sensation of their own clothing. There's a well-known autistic person named Temple Grandin who overcame her own autism to become an accomplished veterinarian and writer. She writes of her own experience as an autistic person. What she writes is, "Loud noises were also a problem, often feeling like a dentist's drill hitting a nerve.

They actually caused pain. I was scared to death of balloons popping, minor noises that most people can tune out drove me to distraction. My roommate's hair dryer sounded like a jet plan taking off." So that's a description of autism from someone who has recovered well enough to write books about it. Another person, L.H. Willey, who has Asperger's syndrome has written, "I found it impossible even to touch some objects. I hated stiff things, satiny things. Goosebumps and chills, and a general sense of unease would follow." So there are wide reports of perceptual difficulties in autistic persons, and that's interesting. It's not obvious why those things would go with the social deficit.

The perceptual deficits by themselves are not a big deal. After all, if perceptual deficits were the only problem that autistics and Asperger's sufferers had, then they would be functional in society. We would just think of these people as eccentrics. But it's possible that these perceptual problems might have a deeper meaning. Recent studies have shown that these perceptual problems show up very early even in toddlers, even in two-year-olds. There have been some very interesting studies that show that autistic kids show possible perceptual problems with biological motion. This is important because biological motion is a means by which we identify persons in our environment as opposed to inanimate objects. There was a study that was done examining biological motion in two-year-olds.

This study was done on biological motion in two-year-olds and this was done with two-year-old autistic children, also typically developing toddlers, and developmentally-delayed toddlers, and that third group is used as a control group. This study is done by attaching lights to a person and taping that person interacting with the doll, playing with the doll saying, look at the doll, and they're taped at a color such that you can only see the lights. So this is often done in movies to capture motion. The experiment is as follows: What's done here is that kids are played the soundtrack that goes with this movie and they're played the dot pattern that goes with the movie. They're also played the same dot pattern upside down and backwards. What happens here is quite striking. If you look at the eye position of where these children are looking, the typical kids, the autistic kids, these two groups have very different patterns of looking. The typical kids spend nearly all of their time looking at the dot pattern that goes with the soundtrack in a right-side up orientation. But the autistic kids don't really make a distinction. If we watch this we can see that difference if we just watch it for awhile. So watch the eye position which is represented by the red plusses, and watch it for the typical toddlers, and watch it for the autistic toddlers as well.

What's going on in this movie then if you look carefully, is that the typical toddlers spend their time looking at the right-side up movie which goes with the soundtrack, as opposed to the autistic kids who seem to not really tell the difference. So what this suggests is that it's not a consequence of developmental delay in general because kids who have a social model seem to have no problem detecting which movie goes with the appropriate soundtrack.

This is interesting because one can detect perceptual problems in autistic children also in other aspects of life. So here's an example. Autistic children when listening to grown-ups who are talking to them, don't look at the eyes. Kids typically look at the eyes of a grown-up who's talking, but autistic kids look at the mouth. It's as if they're really interested in that synchronization of mouth and voice, but in some sense they can't see the social content. This phenomenon suggests the possibility that that perceptual problem is preventing autistic children from getting social cues in the first place. What's interesting about this perceptual problem is that it could be closely associated with the social deficits.

In fact, one attractive possibility is that these perceptual problems might even be a root cause that makes it difficult for babies and children to form social bonds. Imagine if you were born and you couldn't tell when something socially surprising or socially interesting happened. Imagine if you were just deprived of social input. Recall I've talked about children deprived of input such as in the Romanian orphanages. Children who are deprived of social input from a very early age do not form normal social bonds, do not form normal social capacities. So it's attractive to imagine that maybe, perhaps, these perceptual deficits could be the cause of the other social deficits. So that's an attractive possibility.

Another possibility is that perceptual dysfunction and empathetic social deficits may share some common developmental cause. Another possibility is that there's some upstream cause in development that's important in generating both of these capacities. That would be another possibility.

I'm very interested in this idea that perception of salient and unusual events may play an integral role in the form of theory of mind capacity in the first place. I'm very interested in that. Imagine if you couldn't tell whether a moving object were a person or a tree, you would perhaps not be able to form a mental model in which persons and trees were in separate categories. Recall that I said that one of the core abilities of infants at the age of three months was that they're able to tell objects from agents. So it's possible to imagine that this is a problem.

There are other examples of perceptual problems in autistics. For instance, it's commonly observed that if I were to ask you to erase a board, if you were to do that a typical person would go like this and pantomime erasing the board. That would be a fairly typical thing. What an autistic person typically does is find a flat surface, any flat surface, and then make a motion of rubbing that surface. So autistic persons are very concrete in the way they deal with perceptions. Another example is if you ask an autistic person to imagine opening a door by putting a key in a keyhole, I would demonstrate such a thing by taking an imaginary key and going like this and turning. But an autistic person looks for some hole, looks for some aperture like a coffee cup or something, and then goes like this and makes a motion of putting a key in a keyhole. So autistic persons seem to require that kind of tactile feedback and there seems to be some difficulty somewhere in their imagining of that process perhaps imagining the perception. So there's something going on there.

Let's now turn to brain deficits. Let's ask the question, are there places in the brain where deficits are visible anatomically either at the gross level or when you look at cells? It turns out that there are interesting overlaps with what's known about various brain functions. So one place where deficits are visible anatomically in the brains of autistic persons examined postmortem is in the amygdala. I've talked about the amygdala before as being important in processing emotional states of others and also in generating emotional responses. Remember I talked about fear, anxiety, and also positive emotions, and so the amygdala is a site of neuroanatomical abnormality.

Another region that is commonly affected in autistic persons is the cerebellum, and this is interesting. The cerebellum is the most commonly affected brain structure in autistic persons examined at the cellular level. If you look on a microscope slide you will almost always see some deficits in the cerebellum. That's interesting because if you look in medical textbooks or standard textbooks about the brain, what these textbooks say is that the cerebellum is primarily thought of as a brain structure that regulates movement. But it turns out that recent research has suggested that the cerebellum has a more general function. It seems to be important for detecting unexpected events. For instance there are differences in brain activation when another person touches you versus when you touch yourself. So for instance you can't tickle yourself, and if you go like this, that doesn't tickle. But if someone else does it then perhaps it does tickle. So that's an example of a function that appears to involve the cerebellum or that has been suggested to involve the cerebellum. There seems to be some capacity that the cerebellum engages in where it in general seems to be good at detecting unexpected events. This is a major model of cerebellar function that's currently the focus of a lot of research.

I've mentioned the amygdala. I've mentioned the cerebellum. These are areas that have been demonstrated consistently to show differences between autistics and typicals. You might be surprised that I haven't mentioned the neocortex. The neocortex which, after all, is three-fourths of our brain, especially since the insula is part of the cortex and these mirror neurons that I mentioned are also found in the neocortex. So why is it that these have not been mentioned? One possibility is that mirror neurons are, in fact, not that common. You have to search around in the brain to find a mirror neuron. Another possibility is that the deficits in neocortex are, in fact, rather subtle and people have not figured out the right way to examine brain structures in the neocortex to find out what's different in autistic person's brains. So that's one big possibility and I think that's a fairly significant possibility.

Another possibility of course is that these big anatomical deficits that I've described in the amygdala and the cerebellum, it's possible that those deficits are secondary. This is an active area of research and I'll give you my interpretation of this. I favor the idea that these older brain structures, such as the amygdala and the cerebellum, these evolutionarily old structures, play a key role in guiding the development of many characteristics in our brains including ones that are special to us as humans. The amygdala is present in all mammals, the cerebellum is present in all vertebrates, not just mammals, so it's possible, I suggest, that these old brain structures present in all mammals act as teachers to the rest of the brain. Perhaps they act as detectors that say, that's an interesting event, that's a biological object, that's a socially interesting object. So it's possible that these brain structures play a critical role in guiding the brain in its development of theory of mind.

Now let's summarize what we've learned about theory of mind by looking at autism. Autism is a neurological disorder that's marked by an absence of theory of mind. It's associated with problems not only of social interaction, but also problems of perception of the physical and social world. Brain regions that are affected in autism so far to date include the cerebellum and the amygdala. There has also been speculation on particular neocortical areas, without evidence yet, but some speculation about the insular cortex and also mirror neurons.

I've presented to you what's known about autism, what's known about theory of mind. But there's something I haven't covered, and the thing I haven't covered, because it hasn't been done yet, is how it all fits together. One of the central challenges in neuroscience research in general is to understand different levels of function, understanding how molecules work together to generate functional synapses, how neurons talk with one another, how systems of circuits work together, how the whole shebang works together to make a working brain. Another aspect of what's currently a very active area of research is how developmental processes coordinate these brain regions to work separately and together over development and throughout life to generate our many capacities, and in the case of today's lecture, the ability to think about the motivations of other people. Autism is an active area of research both for its medical important, but also at a fundamental level in understanding how these processes develop and in the case of autism, how they can go wrong. So a very active area of research now is to look at the gene mutations that seem to be connected with autism and to look at those gene mutations and see how function is affected in humans or in animals. In particular a very exciting area for the future would be to look for social deficits or perhaps perceptual deficits in animals that have these mutations that are found in us.

In the next lecture what I'd like to do is shift away from the social mind in general. Now in the next lecture I'd like to start talking about sex differences between men and women.

Mars and Venus—Men's and Women's Brains
Lecture 30

The influence of the hypothalamus suggests a way for our brains to be connected to various phenomena that we think of as being separate from our mental processes.

B rain development is under the control of hormones; in the case of differences between the genders, these are sex hormones called **androgens** (male) and **estrogens** (female). Of course, as most of us know, men also make estrogens and women make androgens. These hormones are synthesized by cholesterol and converted by an enzymatic pathway to progesterone and then to testosterone. This chemical pathway shows that, in fact, these sex hormones are shared between men and women. Around the time of birth, sex hormones organize the brain by controlling the development of regions that will eventually become important for sexual behavior. During and after puberty, these behaviors are expressed by male and female hormones acting again.

In the brain, the hypothalamus activates the release of sex hormones in the pituitary. This is interesting because there is neocortical input to the hypothalamus, which means that psychological factors can influence fertility. In women, these hormones orchestrate the 28-day cycle, for example. The influence of the hypothalamus suggests that our brains are connected to various phenomena that we think of as being separate from our mental processes. There is some speculation that androgens and estrogens that increase in puberty might play a role in the mood and psychiatric disorders that appear at that time.

One area of gender differences that is perhaps the most politically fraught is cognitive abilities. Cognitive test performance measures, such as standardized examinations, demonstrate that math and verbal skills are, in fact, similar overall between men and women. This is true of a wide range of performance measures with a few exceptions. The only reliably measured difference between men and women is in manipulations having to do with space: spatial reasoning, memory, and navigation. When it comes to navigation, men tend to be oriented around the coordinates and women are oriented around landmarks.

Another area of contrast is that women tend to have significantly better spatial memory than men. Women are rather good at knowing where things are. The converse of that is in the mental rotation of objects, which is an area where men tend to do better than women. Some of this difference arises as a result of sex hormones acting throughout development, but some of it also happens in adulthood. For instance, amazingly, one shot of testosterone can improve female performance on an object rotation test.

One area of gender differences that is perhaps the most politically fraught is cognitive abilities.

The biggest cognitive difference between men and women is how they deal with spatial reasoning and spatial objects—how they deal with space. In addition, men and women differ in the frequency of neurological and psychiatric disorders. This phenomenon suggests that perhaps the normal ranges for men and women are somewhat different, and when we fall off the end of the range, we fall off in different ways. ∎

Important Terms

androgens: A class of steroid hormones, including testosterone, with roles in aggression and sexual behavior in both sexes but most notably in males.

estrogen: A class of female reproductive hormones.

Questions to Consider

1. How do men and women differ in the way in which they deal with spatial relationships?

2. Are there any other significant gender differences in cognitive ability or mood?

Mars and Venus—Men's and Women's Brains
Lecture 30—Transcript

Welcome back. In the last few lectures we've heard about functions such as personality, intelligence, and how our brain generates social feelings and social constructions. Now what I'd like to do in the next couple of lectures is get into a subject that virtually everyone is interested in which is sex and sex differences. These are subjects that are very easy to persuade people to be interested in. What I'd like to do today is to take that naturally interesting subject and turn it into something a little bit scholarly, but still with the hope of making it useful for your everyday life, something to help you think about a little bit. That'll be the subject of the next two lectures. In this lecture we're going to talk about sex differences, and in the next lecture we're going to talk more about sex itself and about love and pair bonding and how we form bonds with one another.

In this lecture, as I said we're going to talk about sex differences, and so this will begin our brief detour to Mars and Venus. There's a general question that comes up a lot which is, are the sexes different? Obviously this is a politically fraught question in some cases and the answers turn out to be a mix of biology and culture. Some differences are innate and others are imposed upon us or built out of our experience in everyday life as we grow up in whatever country or whatever culture we grow up in.

One surprising answer to many questions about sex differences is that surprisingly we're not all that different, including some ways in which you would, in fact, think that we differ. And so there are many more similarities than differences. In fact, in most areas men and women cover overlapping ranges so that gender is, in fact, only a weak predictor of individual capability. That's true for many things, not all things. So what I thought I'd do today is talk about biological mechanisms, talk about differences that arise early in development near birth and continue through childhood, adolescence, and adulthood. These span a number of areas including mood, cognitive abilities, and neurological and psychiatric disorders.

So as I said, it's not surprising that there are some differences. After all, brain development is under the control of hormones, and in particular in this case sex hormones. Previously we've heard about one kind of hormone, a steroid hormone called "glucocorticoids." These are stress hormones that are in the general category of catabolic hormones, catabolic steroids, meaning in the business of breaking things down. Today our main focus is going to be sex hormones which are in the category of anabolic steroids which are in the business of building up. For instance, examples of anabolic steroids, sex hormones, include estrogen, estradiol, and testosterone. These sex hormones have different effects on the body including the building of secondary sex characteristics and they also have influences on the brain.

The most dramatic sex differences in the entire brain are found on the parts that contribute to what you do in bed, or what you would like to be doing in bed. These sexual behavior areas of the brain show large enough differences that you can tell whether a particular brain is male or female just by looking at those regions. As it turns out, those sex differences begin to develop before birth, despite the fact that they don't get used until later. Here's how it all begins. Male and female brains start developing and differentiating from one another during brain development from an origin that's genetically determined. There's a gene that's on the male specific Y chromosome, so remember that the Y chromosome is only found in males, and X chromosomes are found one in males and then two in females. There's a gene on the Y chromosome that directs the production of a factor that induces formation of testicles in male fetuses, and so male fetuses develop testicles in response to this particular gene. The testicles then release testosterone, one of these sex hormones, to promote specific changes in the brain and the sex organs. These specific changes are male-specific and so therefore these changes are called "masculinization." Also, testosterone directs the secretion of other hormones to suppress the development of female sex organs, and so there's this push-pull phenomenon which some things get turned on, other things get turned off.

One thing that's interesting about the development of brain and body structures is that female sexual development doesn't require any hormones at this very early stage. So what appears to be the case is that in development, the program of setting up the body and brain seems to have a default mode in which in the absence of additional hormone the default sex is female. Then testosterone is added to force events to move towards maleness.

These sex hormones act in two major stages during development. The first stage is around the time of birth. Around the time of birth sex hormones organize the brain by controlling the development of regions that will eventually become important for sexual behavior. Even though those regions are obviously not used at that time, they're setup at that time. These behaviors are not expressed until they're activated after puberty, during and after puberty, by male and female hormones acting again. Both stages around birth and at puberty must be successful for normal sexual behavior to occur. Now let's take a look at how these sex hormones are made in the body.

Sex hormones are made starting from the chemical cholesterol. We often hear about cholesterol as being a bad chemical, but in fact cholesterol is necessary for the synthesis of sex hormones. So cholesterol synthesized is converted by an enzymatic pathway to progesterone and then to testosterone. Testosterone is the first of the male hormones and so male hormones are generally called "androgens." Then through a second step, testosterone is converted by an enzyme called "aromatase" to another hormone called "estradiol," and estradiol is an example of an estrogen. So female hormones are estradiol and progesterone. This is a pathway in which these chemicals are converted one to the other by the addition or conversion of chemical bonds. What you end up with is a synthesis that's in a sequential pathway. Because of the sequential pathway, what that means is that in fact in addition to male hormones, men also make estrogens, and conversely women make androgens. It's just that men have more androgens and women have more estrogens. This pathway shows us that, in fact, these sex hormones are shared between men and women.

How are these sex hormones secreted? We've talked about the hypothalamus a lot with regard to other functions, in particular emotional responses and also stress responses. Now the hypothalamus strikes again, this little region that's the size of a large grape turns out to also be deeply involved in sexual maturation and also in sexual behavior.

In this case the hypothalamus, we begin at the hypothalamus, and in this case now what happens is that the hypothalamus releases something called "gonadotropin releasing hormone." This gonadotropin releasing hormone, in fact, has the job of releasing gonadotropin. These are easy things to remember. GNRH, as it's called, is released by the hypothalamus and then it's detected by the anterior pituitary. Again it's the hypothalamus, then the pituitary, something that we've heard about before. Now what happens is the pituitary then releases gonadotropins. Gonadotropins are hormones that are particularly important for normal sexual development and function in both women and men. There are several major gonadotropins that turn up a lot, one is something that is called "luteinizing hormone," or just "LH" for short, and another one is called "follicle stimulating hormones," called "FSH" for short. In this case follicle stimulating hormone has the job of going to follicles, and in this case they are the testes or the ovaries.

Let's now think a little bit about what these gonadotropins do to the gonads, to the testes and ovaries. LH and FSH influence sperm development. LH specifically triggers testes to make testosterone, and testosterone and FSH, the other gonadotropin I mentioned, are involved in the maturation of sperm. This is interesting both because it's brain-directed sperm maturation, and in particular what's interesting to note here is that there is, of course, neocortical input to the hypothalamus. The neocortex influences the hypothalamus, and we've talked about that. What that means is that psychological factors can, in fact, influence fertility. In females these hormones orchestrate the 28-day monthly cycle. That is associated with the fact that in fact, for instance, women who live together often synchronize their 28-day monthly cycles. The fact that neocortex influences hypothalamus provides one way in which this could happen. So the fact that the brain influences the hypothalamus suggests a way for our brains to be connected to these various phenomena that we think of as being separate from our mental processes.

Now let's back up a little bit. We were on the subject of early development, let's talk more about testosterone and brain development. I referred to Stage 1 and Stage 2. Let's go back to Stage 1. In Stage 1, testosterone produced by the testes during a critical period around birth leads to initial masculinization of the brain, and also leads to male-typical behaviors. I will come back to what these male-typical behaviors are later. I'll give you one example right now, an example of a male-typical behavior is rough and tumble play which is seen in human children and also in mammalian pups. I should note that when testosterone has these effects—this is a little complicated, but I'll make the note right now—when testosterone acts upon the brain, there's something that's perhaps counter to expectation which is that I showed you that chemical pathway in which testosterone can be made to estradiol. It turns out that for testosterone at this stage of development to have an effect on the brain, and in particular to direct the formation of male behaviors, it goes into the brain and it's converted by that enzyme aromatase to estradiol. It's the hormone estradiol which we think of as a female sex hormone that in fact directs masculinization of the brain, and so there's a little irony there and it's a detail that's a little funny.

Now let's fast forward a little bit past childhood and go to puberty. These same hormones have actions on the brain and on the body during puberty. In addition to the direction and the activation of these brain regions that I mentioned before, these hormones also have effects on the body. For example, in males, testosterone leads to increased muscular development and in the growth of facial hair. In females estrogens rise during puberty and lead to the maturation of their reproductive systems and in particular also lead to the development of breasts, the growth of breasts.

These hormones in adults, let's talk about adult everyday life, these hormones vary throughout one's everyday life. Let's talk about men for a moment. Men have about 10 times the level of testosterone as women on average overall. But in men that level in fact is not constant. It varies during the day. It varies in response to experiences. For example, testosterone levels are higher in cases of social challenge or anger or conflict. These are situations in which testosterone rises. Testosterone rises when men think about sex, when men anticipate sex. Those are conditions in which testosterone levels go up. There are some other interesting details that have been found. One detail is that if you're a sports fan and your team wins, then your testosterone levels go up. So your team winning is, in some sense, overlapping in your brain with thinking about sex. When your team loses, testosterone levels go down. Testosterone levels, in short, go up and down in response to daily events that are associated not only with sex, but also with aggression, and also action.

In women, estrogens take longer to cycle than testosterone. In women that cycle is, as of course you can guess, 28-days long. So in women these sex hormones cycle, but in fact with a 28-day period as it were. So let's talk a little bit about these cyclings. So the main lesson here is that testosterone cycles much more quickly than estrogens. People often talk about premenstrual syndrome, the idea that somehow you're in a worse mood or a different mood depending on what point a woman is in her cycle. I would present that perhaps there is this other kind of thing that's not talked about, what one could perhaps call non-menstrual syndrome. I remember it when I was younger and frankly moodier, I used to have ups and down in my mood and I used to tell people, as a joke, that I had non-menstrual syndrome. And so one can, in fact, detect these mood changes that are probably connected with hormonal changes.

I mentioned early in this lecture that in the adult brain there are anatomical differences, but not that many. There are some nervous differences that turn up here or there. So for instance there's a particular nucleus of the hypothalamus that's larger in men than in women. If you look in rats you can find a particular cluster of neurons that's larger in one sex than in the other. But overall what's surprising perhaps is that there are not that many differences between male and female brains, despite the fact that there are these changes of course in behavior and in things like partner preference. So what appears to be the case is that the subtleties in the differences in brain function evidently must arise from features that are too subtle to see when looking at gross brain structures. So even though there are sex differences, it's not necessarily the case that we can look at a brain and see what is the underlying cause of those sex differences in behavior.

Certainly brains of both sexes have mechanisms for receiving sex hormones, so sex hormones act upon the brain. You can find sex hormone receptors, so these molecules that bind to the sex hormones throughout the brain. In particular you can find them in high density in deep core brain regions, regions that include of course the hypothalamus and pituitary. They themselves receive back sex hormones and have receptors that the hormones can bind to. In addition you can find sex hormone receptors in the preoptic area, also in the midbrain in core brain structures, as well as in the hippocampus, and in other brain regions.

Estrogen receptors, let's take estrogen receptors in particular, have multiple kinds of receptors and those receptors can response either very quickly or more slowly to estrogen. So, for example, estrogen receptors are found on synaptic vesicles and synaptic vesicles can, in fact, even be moved within presynaptic terminals, the structures that release neurotransmitter, in response to estrogen. That's an example of a fast action. Estrogen can also bind to neurotransmitter receptors and alter the action of neurotransmitter receptors. So these are all examples of things that estrogen can do quickly. Estrogen also acts upon receptors that are in the nucleus. Recall that the nucleus is where the DNA is found and that's where DNA is copied to make RNA. It turns out that estrogen can bind to direct the transcription of DNA to be copied into RNA. So estrogen can, in fact, direct the output of cells as they make RNA and then to make protein.

As a result of these mechanisms for estrogen action on the brain, it's possible to see changes in neurons in response to estrogen and I'll give you an example. These effects can actually be quite large. For instance during a female rat's 5-day estrus cycle, hippocampal neurons sprout like mad when estrogen is high. You can see the difference in looking at these dendrites at high and low points of estrogen in a rat's cycle. This was worked on at Rockefeller University by Bruce McEwen, Liz Gould, and Catherine Woolley, and this has been followed up by them in the years since then. You can see these things on the hippocampal dendrites. It turns out that they're excitatory connections, so they are connections that excite these neurons. In fact what has been observed is that rats are more susceptible to seizures at times when these spines have sprouted. So that's an example of estrogen acting upon the brain in a fairly direct sort of way in which you can see what's happening at a single-cell level.

Now let's talk a little bit about adult function. I talked about, mostly jokingly, about mood swings in men and women. There is a popular belief. The popular belief is that women are moodier than men. It is true that women are moody. What most people don't realize is that men are moody too, as I referred to in my own moods. It turns out that when this is carefully studied men's moods vary as much from hour to hour as women's moods. So for example, a study has been done in which psychologists give beepers to men and women and ask them to write down their mood every time the beeper goes off. What's observed is that men and women report similar variations in their mood. They're both equally variable in their moods.

What's curious is that even though they're equally moody, both men and women tend to remember women's mood swings better. So if people are asked later to remember how moody they or their partners were in the previous week, more mood swings are reported for women than men. What appears to be the case is that even though we're both as moody as one another, women's moods are somehow more memorable to everyone. So that appears to be near the core of this popular belief.

I've talked about the fact that sex hormones start affecting the brain around birth, and in fact it is possible to see behavioral differences between boys and girls quite early in life. They start emerging early in childhood. One example is in the case of toy preference. One often encounters, when looking at little boys and little girls, no matter how hard you try it is very hard to dissuade children from their natural toy preference, whatever it might be. I have one colleague who has multiple children, she has a boy and a girl, and one thing she did at one point was to try to break down this toy preference. She took a doll and gave it to the boy and she gave two trucks to the girl. She later found, to her surprise, and perhaps a little bit of horror, that she found the boy using the doll to attempt to pound a nail. She also found the girl with the trucks and rather than going vroom, vroom with the trucks, she had the two trucks next to each other and they were kissing one another. So these preferences are sometimes really well ingrained in us. I should say that these toy preferences do appear to be affected by sex hormones. This is true in rhesus monkeys for instance. It's possible to influence behavior early in life by altering sex hormone signaling in rats and in rhesus monkeys. Here's an example.

If a genetic female, either rat or rhesus monkey, is treated with androgens during critical periods of prenatal development or neonatal development, they will show increased rough and tumble play. In humans this happens before birth. In the case of androgen treatment, human children also develop an interest in having male playmates, an interest in boy-type toys like trucks and balls, and a reduced interest in girl-type toys. That's fairly typical, and these are preferences that typically show up at the end of infancy and you can see it very easily in our one- or two-year-olds. As I've mentioned, for boys this appears to be things like construction and transportation tools, and in girls it appears to be more human-oriented social toys such as dolls.

Girls with a genetic disorder, so like the rats and the monkeys, in us, in girls with a genetic disorder that exposes them to high levels of testosterone and other androgens before birth, again they are more interested in toy trucks and cars than typical girls are. There are other differences as well. One difference is a smaller one. I mentioned rough and tumble play. That difference is, again, apparent between boys and girls, but the interest in rough and tumble play is fairly small between boys and girls. It's not nearly so large as this difference in toy preference. However, these changes, whether large or small, are likely to be reinforced by play because recall that I mentioned that children prefer compatible play styles and they tend to pick playmates of the same sex. So little girls will tend to pick one another to play with, and what that means is that whatever innate tendency there is, whether small or large, would be likely to be reinforced by simple repetition, just the learning of experience.

We can ask how do we know whether these toy preferences are innate? How do we know that they're not perhaps culturally imposed from the beginning? One piece of evidence comes from a study done on vervet monkeys. It turns out that very young vervet monkeys have been given toys and the kinds of toys they've been given include a police car and a ball and a doll, and they in fact also have gender-specific preferences. For example, if you look at pictures of baby vervet monkeys playing with the toys in this study. You can find a female vervet monkey examining a doll and doing an anogenital inspection of the doll the way that they would do with, in fact, a live primate of their own species. You can see a young male monkey of the species taking a truck and going vroom, vroom with the truck. These are things that you can see, and there are significant preference differences where the males tend to like the truck and the females tend to like the doll.

This leads to the possible speculation that males perhaps have innate evolved preferences for objects that involve movement, and perhaps females might have innate preferences, say for socially oriented objects. I should say that there's no clear preference between these two for other objects that seem to be neutral, books and stuffed animals appear to be well liked by both males and females in vervet monkeys, as is the case in us.

I've talked about mood. I said that mood is something that seems to be similarly variable in women and men, we're as moody as one another. But

I also said—recall that I said in a previous lecture—that many psychiatric disorders start turning up around puberty. That's the time when androgens and estrogens start working on the brain. So it's not clear why or how, but it's possible that those hormones could possibly play a role, and here are some examples. Although moods vary similarly between women and men, mood disorders are a different story. Mood disorders including depression and anxiety are about twice as common in women as in men. Some of that may be due to the fact that women are more willing to go the doctor when they feel bad, but even when we account for cultural difference, it appears that women are still at greater risk for these mood disorders. It's not clear why that is, but one possibility is that women's life experiences, since they're smaller and also less prone to aggression, more likely to perhaps be the objects of aggression, perhaps their life experiences may expose them to more stress which is linked to depression and anxiety. This is not true of all psychiatric disorders. For example, men and women are equally prone to manic-depressive disorder which has a genetic component, but is not sex specific. So these are examples of ways in which mood disorders can vary between the sexes.

Another case is autism, and it's not clear why, but the difference is in the converse direction. More men, more boys, are autistic than women and girls. This is again unclear why. It has been suggested that autism represents the endpoint of a personality range that is typically male. For instance, we talked about males having more of an interest in objects rather than people. It's possible, and it has been suggested by an autism researcher Simon Baron-Cohen, that there is a range of personality traits that you can find in boys, perhaps they're more variable than in girls, and that range includes variable interests in objects. If you go to the endpoint of this natural tendency, perhaps these innate tendencies start to become difficult for everyday life and turn into autism once you get to the endpoint of the range. So that has been suggested as a possible reason for why it is that males are more likely to be autistic or have autistic spectrum disorder than females.

We've talked about mood; we've talked about personality and psychiatric disorders. One area that is perhaps the most politically fraught is cognitive abilities, the ability to think, to solve problems. What's really remarkable in this area I should say, before I get into the evidence, is that women and men are remarkably not that different in many respects and this is interesting. Let's first start by considering the neocortex, the part of the brain that we value for its cognitive abilities, and let's just look at the gross structure. In women, brains tend to have more surface area and more connections between different distant areas. So these are features of women's brains compared with men's brains. Men's brains tend to be larger, they tend to have more volume, even when you correct for body size. So a man and a woman of the same body weight will have slightly different brains on average, where the men will have slightly larger brains than the women.

This difference is tiny compared with some other animals. It's possible to find differences between males and females in the brains of nearly every species, but in fact, in other species the differences are often quite large. In an extreme example, in gorillas, males have much larger bodies and their brains are twice as large as females, so in gorillas there's a tremendous difference. Back to our species, in our species these differences are small. And if you look at cognitive test performance measures such as standardized examinations, what's found is that math and verbal skills are, in fact, similar overall. The averages are the same and sometimes you can see an isolated report in the literature of some difference, but overall there seems to be very little difference in test performance between men and women. This is true of a wide range of performance measures with a few exceptions, and the exceptions are as follows. The only reliably measured difference between men and women is in manipulations having to do with space, spatial reasoning, memory, and navigation. Let's go through that a little bit.

When it comes to navigation, men tend to be oriented around coordinates and women are oriented around landmarks. I'll give you an example. I'll start with animals again. I'll start with rats. You can put a rat in an arena with local landmarks to navigate around, and also distant landmarks like painting on the walls or pictures on the wall. If you rotate the arena and ask the male to navigate some more, this male rat will make more errors than the female rats. On the other hand, female rates will make more errors if you change the local landmarks and are less oriented towards the distant pictures on the wall or what have you. So in us if you hear the phrase, the direction of something like go past the stone church on the left and then turn right a few blocks later at the tan house with the big tan tree, you're probably listening to a women.

If you hear go south for 1.6 miles then go east for another half mile, then the odds are that it's a man talking.

So another area of contrast is that women tend to be very good at spatial memory. So this is a large difference between men and women. Women are rather good at knowing where things are. For instance, if there's a bunch of objects that you show to a woman and say which one moved, the average women is better than about 80 percent of men. So that's an area in which spatial memory is different between the sexes, in this case women do somewhat better. The converse of that is in the mental rotation of objects. Here's an area where men tend to do better than women. If you show an object rotation problem, for instance if you say, okay look at this cube pattern, and ask which of these three comparison shapes is the same object except rotated, that performance difference is rather large. Men, on average, do much better on this than women. The average man performs better than on this than about 80 percent of women. It's a fairly significant difference and you can see it in individuals that you might meet.

Some of this arises through sex hormones acting throughout development, but some of it also happens in adulthood. For instance, amazingly, one shot of testosterone can improve female performance on this test. One colleague I have is a developmental neuroscientist who began life as a woman, and when she was a woman she decided to get a sex change and she took this test at one point and found it rather hard and had to mentally manipulate the object and turn it around slowly in order to figure out what the answer was. Then as she got testosterone treatments it became easier and easier and she got shot after shot, and eventually he found that it was actually a natural and easy task. So that's possible to change even in adult life.

Finally I want to address what I would call "the Lawrence Summers problem," and I'll get to why that is. That's the problem of extreme scientific abilities. Summers is an economist by trade. He was asked to speak while he was president of Harvard to a conference on the subject of why women were underrepresented in the highest reaches of science. He went into a speculation about why it was that men were more likely to have very high scores on standardized tests despite the fact that the averages were the same. He listed a few possibilities. One possibility he listed was perhaps the differences are innate. His expertise is in economics, not in neuroscience, and he was speaking in his capacity as a university president and it's perhaps not surprising that shortly after that he was no longer president of Harvard University.

What's interesting to note here is despite the fact that there's this difference between male and female performance at the very highest levels of these tests, that's changed. That gap has closed significantly. For instance, if we take the math portion of the Scholastic Aptitude Test, the SAT, the gender ratio of kids scoring above 700, between 700 and 800 on that test, used to be 12 to 1, 12 times as many boys as girls got over 700 on that, and that was in 1982. But by the late 1990s that ratio had closed from 12 to 1 to 3 to 1, and that's a really large change to happen in just a few decades. What that suggests is that these gender inequities perhaps are not innate. Perhaps the abolishment of gender inequities in society, the reduction in inequities, can help the most able students and all students really, to perform better on this examination and to perform better in society.

What have we learned today? We've learned that despite differences in hormone- dependent maturation along the way, women's and men's brains in many ways are surprisingly similar and they remain sensitive to sex hormones not only throughout development and puberty, but even in adult life. In adult life many measures between men and women are the same or similar to one another: mood variation, problem solving in most areas, and most intelligence tests. The biggest cognitive difference between men and women is how they deal with spatial reasoning and spatial objects, how they deal with space. In addition to this, men and women differ in the frequency of neurological and psychiatric disorders. In this case what the phenomenon suggests is that perhaps the normal ranges for men and women are somewhat different, and so when we fall off the end of the range, we fall off in different ways.

I've talked about all these differences, but I think that this is going to be an area of active research for a long time in the future. I'll conclude by quoting the humorist Robert Orben who said, "Nobody will ever win the battle of the sexes, there's too much fraternization with the enemy."

In the next lecture we will talk about sex per se, and we will talk about love and partnership.

Sex, Love, and Bonds for Life
Lecture 31

When we look at what happens during sexual behavior, it turns out
... the neural pathways that lead to sexual behavior ... involve quite
similar neural circuits. ... In that respect, we're quite similar.

When we look at what happens during sexual behavior, the mechanics of sex—and by mechanics, we mean the neural pathways that lead to sexual behavior in men and women—involve quite similar neural circuits. Sexual performance requires the **sympathetic** and **parasympathetic nervous systems**, which push and pull our behavior in ways that are related to the stress system. What this means is that sexual performance is connected with the stress response. Stress has chronic effects on sexual behavior—for instance, in women, irregular menstrual cycles or even the cessation of menses and, in men, decreased sperm count and testosterone levels. For both men and women, interest in sexual behavior decreases with stress. Under conditions of stress, men often report problems with erections.

Orgasm itself has been imaged by Dutch scientists, who have found that the brain's reward system is activated during orgasm in both sexes, but there are differences between men and women. Women showed reduced activity in an area of the frontal cortex that might relate to a reduction of inhibition. Men showed reduced activity in the amygdala, where fear, anxiety, and vigilance arise. That suggests that during orgasm, men might experience a reduction in vigilance. Men and women shared increased activity in the cerebellum. The cerebellum has been implicated in emotional arousal and in sensory surprise, reflecting its role in reporting unexpected events.

One of the few reliable sex differences has been found in one particular area of the human hypothalamus, the third interstitial nucleus, which is twice as large in men as in women. A neuroscientist who has studied this nucleus in straight men and in gay men found that it was about half as large in gay men as in straight men. Although it's not at all known how this nucleus might be involved in generating sexual orientation, the fact that we can see these differences at all suggests the possibility of understanding preference as a biological mechanism.

Turning to the phenomenon of love, studies in voles have offered insight into how we form partnerships. In voles, the mechanism by which bonding occurs relies on vasopressin and **oxytocin**—major neuromodulator peptides made in the hypothalamus. They're also made in the ovaries or testes, and they play a critical role in pair bond formation. In the prairie vole, oxytocin released into the brain of a female during sexual activity is important for forming a monogamous pair bond with her sexual partner. Vasopressin appears to have a similar effect in males.

The cerebellum has been implicated in emotional arousal and in sensory surprise, reflecting its role in reporting unexpected events.

Returning to humans, during orgasm in women, oxytocin levels increase, and during sexual arousal in men, vasopressin concentrations increase. In addition, imaging experiments during romantic love show activation of reward areas, particularly regions that have receptors for oxytocin and vasopressin. These findings suggest that romantic love in humans and partnered pair bonding may involve oxytocin, vasopressin, and the brain's reward circuitry. The brain's reward areas, in the context of dopamine and addiction, are involved in the formation of addiction and in the signaling of reward. This suggests that release of dopamine may be critical for the response to such rewards as food, sex, and addictive drugs. One attractive possibility is that love, in some sense, may be the original addiction. ∎

Important Terms

oxytocin: The "love" molecule; a peptide hormone released by the hypothalamus; plays a role in a number of processes, including "bonding" in social animals.

parasympathetic nervous system: Part of the peripheral autonomic nervous system associated with "rest and digest" functions.

sympathetic nervous system: The part of the peripheral autonomic nervous system involved with the "fight or flight" response.

Questions to Consider

1. What biochemical signals are shared among sexual, familial, and trust-based bonding?

2. Is monogamy the norm or the exception among mammals? Birds?

Sex, Love, and Bonds for Life
Lecture 31—Transcript

Welcome back. In the last lecture, we talked about differences between the sexes—how hormones can direct the development of the nervous system and the body, to lead to differences between males and females. In this lecture, I'd like to examine the counterpart of that which is sexual behavior itself and also love and pair bonding. Today what I'd like to do is talk about the mechanics and neuroscience of sexual behavior. I'll also talk about love, attachment, and in particular the major chemicals that are used by the brain to signal these behavioral phenomena—oxytocin and vasopressin. I'd like to cover how these chemicals are important not only for the feeling of intense romantic attachment, but also for parenting, and even for friendship, trust, and negotiation—all these different things.

When we look at what happens during sexual behavior, it turns out the mechanics of sex—and by "mechanics" I mean the neural mechanics, the neural pathways that lead to sexual behavior, the sex act in men and women—involve quite similar neural circuits. These neural circuits that go through the spinal cord and go to the genitals culminate in increased blood flow in certain parts of external genitals. That's true for both men and women. In that respect, we're quite similar to one another.

Sexual performance requires the sympathetic and parasympathetic nervous systems. Recall some time ago that I talked about the fight, flight, fright, and sex response. That was something that was pioneered, among other people, by Walter Cannon. These sympathetic and parasympathetic nervous systems push and pull our behavior in ways that are related to, of course, the stress system. What this means—the fact that sexual performance requires these same nervous structures—is that sexual performance is connected with the stress response and with the brain's and the nervous system's systems for stress.

Recall in a previous lecture that I mentioned that stress has chronic effects on sexual behavior. For instance, in women, irregular menstrual cycles or even the cessation of menses, and in men, sperm count going down, testosterone levels decreasing. For both men and women, interest in sexual behavior decreases with stress. There are also acute effects, affects that happen right away. Because these behaviors depend on the sympathetic and parasympathetic nervous systems pushing and pulling, what that means is there is an implication for sex. For instance, the parasympathetic nervous system, which principally uses acetylcholine, is responsible for the initiation of sex acts. An example is the engorgement of sexual structures of genitals and lubrications. In males, this includes getting an erection.

The sympathetic nervous system, which uses adrenaline, is responsible for muscular contractions, driving male and female orgasm, and also in males, ejaculations. Under conditions of stress, men often report problems with erections. This is connected with the sympathetic versus the parasympathetic nervous system. It perhaps is surprising that the parasympathetic nervous system, which is typically associated with relaxation, is important for initiating the sex act, for erections. This is opposed to the sympathetic nervous system, which is—in other arenas of behavior—associated with stress and escape. There's a mnemonic that medical students use to understand the role of the parasympathetic and sympathetic nervous systems in the sex act; "P" is for parasympathetic and "S" is for sympathetic. The mnemonic they have is "point and shoot." That makes it easier to remember which of these nervous systems is related to the various parts of the sex act.

Orgasm itself can be imaged. It has been imaged by Dutch scientists who have looked at human brain activity during orgasm by putting people in PET scanners during orgasm. They've seen a number of things. One of them is that, unsurprisingly perhaps, the brain's reward system is activated during orgasm in both sexes. In particular, there are differences between men and women here. What they reported was that women showed reduced activity in an area of the frontal cortex which might relate to a reduction of inhibition. Men showed reduced activity in the amygdala. That suggests, say, for instance, fear, anxiety, vigilance, that perhaps during orgasm there might be a reduction in vigilance in men.

One thing that men and women shared in common is increased activity in the cerebellum. We've talked about the cerebellum before. The cerebellum has been implicated in emotional arousal and also in unexpected sensory events, sensory surprise. Remember, long ago in a lecture on perception, I talked about the cerebellum's role in reporting unexpected events. Evidently this study by the Dutch scientist was studying something that was in that general category.

These are the changes that are associated with the sex act itself, what about sexual orientation? Recall in the last lecture that I mentioned that one of the few reliable sex differences has been found in one particular area of the human hypothalamus. That area is called the "third interstitial nucleus." The hypothalamus, despite being small, is composed of many little clusters of neurons. One of them is this third interstitial nucleus. This nucleus is twice as large in men than in women. There's a neuroscientist, Simon LeVay, who himself is gay, who has studied this particular nucleus in straight men and in gay men. What he has found is that this area was about half as large in gay men as in straight men. In other words, in gay men, this third nucleus was about the size as was found in women. This has not been studied in women to the same level of detail, but in men, this is what he found.

This is hard to interpret in terms of complex behavior. It's not at all known how this nucleus might be involved in generating sexual orientation. But, what's intriguing about it is that it seems to be a first step in understanding something about the biology of how our brains generate sexual preference. The fact that we can see these differences at all suggests the possibility of eventually understanding this kind of preference in terms of a biological mechanism.

That's adult life; now what about early in life? Early in life it is possible to find predictors of homosexuality. It turns out that if you look early in life, the number one predictor of homosexuality in men—that's been detected and studied—is birth order. This is interesting. This is not genetic, but it is something related to your early development. Each older brother increases the odds that a later born male will be gay by 33 percent. Okay, so let's think about what this means. Gay men are probably about 2.5 percent of the male population; that's approximately the case. A boy with one older brother would therefore have not a 2.5 percent chance, but a 3.3 percent chance of growing up to be gay. A boy with two older brothers has a 4.2 percent chance. These are probabilities that are not very high. But, according to these statistics, roughly 15 percent of gay men owe their sexual orientation to the fact that they have older brothers. In contrast, there appears to be no birth order effect on homosexuality and women. Nobody's really sure quite how having older brothers affects sexual orientation, but this is the one thing that's been reported as being a relatively strong effect.

I'd like to turn away from these phenomena to now the phenomenon of love. In particular, I want to talk about love, how we form partnerships, how we decide to form partnerships, whether there's something special about it, and whether we can study it by looking at other mammals. Surprisingly, very few mammals are monogamous. If you look at the ways that mammals mate and form partnerships, only 3 to 5 percent of mammals are monogamous. It is by far the norm in nature for mammals to form temporary alliances, mate, part ways, and not come back together again. That's the standard among mammals. Only 3 to 5 percent of mammals are monogamous. It's somewhat higher in primates; 12 percent of primates are monogamous. In human cultures, they're mostly monogamous. There are exceptions and variations, but the general tendency in human society is to be monogamous. We are among that 12 percent of primates. What's interesting is that there is one group of animals that is mostly monogamous. That's birds. Ninety percent of birds are monogamous. This phenomenon of love birds really is a real phenomenon—not only the species, but also, in general, birds tend to partner for life.

One place where we can study this, then, is in a mammal that's monogamous. Of course, there aren't that many of them. One place where this has been studied quite well and has generated a lot of insight into how partnerships are formed is with voles. Voles are a family of mammals. They come in multiple species. We've learned a lot about how the brain may form bonds from voles. There are different species of voles that have different mating habits. I'll give you the two stars of the story. One star is prairie voles. Prairie voles are in the category of monogamous mammals. Prairie voles mate and they take one mate for life. When mother prairie voles take care of their young, they take care of them and nurture them for an extended period.

I'll contrast those with a close relative of prairie voles; they look very similar, at least to me. I guess that's maybe volist of me. These other voles are montane voles which are similar looking to prairie voles, but they have promiscuous breeding habits. So a typical behavior of montane voles is that a male and a female vole will meet, they'll mate, and then they'll part ways. When female voles raise their young, they spend a little bit of time with their young. As soon as the young are able to, the mothers move on and then the young are packed off.

In these two species of voles, prairie and montane voles, it's possible to measure bonding in the laboratory. What scientists have done is they've allowed voles to wander around in a maze. They've set up a container with three rooms connected by tubes. You have a tube and then the voles in the study can be put in one empty room or another empty room. The vole that's being tested is placed in an empty room. It's connected by two passageways; one room contains the vole's mate and the other contains a stranger. Thus, the vole has a choice between who to spend time with. The more time the vole spends in the room with the mate, the more bonded it is. That's the definition of bonding. Unsurprisingly, the strongest stimulus for the formation of a pair bond between voles is having sex with a partner. When these prairie voles have sex, then they become bonded. Although, it is also true that prairie voles often become bonded simply by living together. The proximity of living with your buddy vole allows you to become friends and to want to spend more time together. That is also the case.

These signals in voles, this mechanism by which this bonding occurs, relies on several major neuromodulator peptides. They are vasopressin and oxytocin. In voles, males make vasopressin and females make oxytocin. In us, we make oxytocin; all of us make oxytocin. These are neuromodulators that are made in the hypothalamus, so we're back to the hypothalamus again. From the hypothalamus, these signals go to the bloodstream. They go to control all kinds of responses including blood vessels, smooth muscle, and also into the brain. These modulators are peptides—oxytocin and arginine vasopressin that's the full name of vasopressin—sometimes when you read the papers, technical and news articles, you see "AVP," which is also vasopressin.

Oxytocin and vasopressin are these little molecules that are nine amino acids long. They're just nine amino acids arranged in a chain. These nine amino acid sequences are different by just two amino acids. Oxytocin and vasopressin are quite similar to one another in structure. They play a critical role in pair bond formation. They're made in the brain and they're also made in the ovaries or testes. One place where they're released is in the pituitary where they can guide many, many outcomes. Oxytocin is released in many mammals during vaginal or cervical stimulation. It's also released during childbirth and mating. So it's released under a variety of conditions relating to sex and the raising of young.

In the prairie vole, oxytocin released into the brain of the female during sexual activity is important for forming a monogamous pair bond with her sexual partner. Vasopressin appears to have a similar effect in males. These molecules appear to be very important in triggering that formation of a bond in prairie voles. Oxytocin—and I'll come back to this in a few minutes—is also important for mother-infant bonding in many species. It seems to be more important for pair bonding in female voles than in males. I talked about oxytocin and vasopressin as being important in pair bonding.

Vasopressin is also important for a variety of male behaviors including aggression. In particular, vasopressin seems to be involved in triggering aggression by one male toward other males. If you imagine pair bonding, you might imagine a part of pair bonding that is not liking the other males. Thus, there is this sort of jealousy-like effect going on there where other males need to keep away.

We can ask, how do we know that these neural systems are important for pair-bond formation? The best evidence for the involvement of these signaling pathways in pair bonding is that it's possible to juice up these pathways to convert the behavior of a promiscuous montane vole to be more like the behavior of the stay-at-home prairie vole. If we look at the brains of prairie and montane voles, you can see differences in the receptors for these molecules. Prairie voles have many more receptors for vasopressin. You can take the vasopressin receptor and, through tools of molecular biology, put the vasopressin receptor into the brain of a promiscuous montane vole. In particular, if you experimentally induce expression of this receptor in the ventral pallidum of one of these promiscuous voles, what you can do is you can get pair bonding to be much stronger. You can convert these promiscuous voles into stay-at-home voles.

What this shows is that a fairly complex behavior like pair bonding can be basically turned on or off by a single gene in a single brain area. Of course, genes in other brain areas are also required. There's a complex set of changes that happens throughout the brain once that switch is flipped. But, the fact of the matter is it's possible to flip that switch experimentally in a vole. One might ask, does the same mechanism apply in humans? Do we use oxytocin and vasopressin? We don't know for sure, but there is some evidence that the idea's plausible. Here are examples of the evidence.

During orgasm in women oxytocin levels increase. That's one example. Another is that, during sexual arousal in men, vasopressin concentrations increase. These are pieces of evidence that there's some connection between us and these voles. In addition, imaging experiments during romantic love—so if you get people who are in the throes of romantic love and you do functional imaging on their brains—you can see that there's activation of reward areas. There's also, as I mentioned before, activation of reward areas in the brain during orgasm. In particular, some of the regions that are activated have receptors for oxytocin and vasopressin. People who are intensely in love show activity in the ventral tegmental area and the caudate. These are parts of the brain's core. After about a year, people in longer-term relationships show activation of other regions including the ventral pallidum. That's the site that I mentioned before as the sight of prairie vole bonding. When people have been together for about a year, they show this activation when they look at a picture of their lover.

These findings suggest that romantic love in humans and also partnered pair bonding may involve oxytocin, vasopressin, and the brain's reward circuitry—all of which are important for pair bonding in voles. Some of these structures are reward structures. We've talked about reward before in the context of dopamine and addition. A possibility that is attractive is that love, in some sense, may be the original addiction. Monogamous prairie voles have more receptors for vasopressin and oxytocin receptors than promiscuous meadow voles in certain key areas. These key areas are involved in the formation of addiction and in the signaling of reward. They include structures in the core of the brain that include the nucleus accumbens, which has lots of oxytocin receptors, and also the ventral pallidum which I've mentioned a few times.

Locally blocking either set of receptors prevents pair bonding as does blocking oxytocin receptors in the prefrontal cortex or blocking vasopressin receptors in the lateral septum of males—another one of these core reward brain structures. What this suggests is that release of dopamine, this reward chemical, may be critical for the response to natural rewards like food, sex, and, as I've mentioned in a previous lecture, addictive drugs.

This idea of love being the original addiction can account for why it is that the brain has pathways devoted for making people crave white powders that never occur naturally. Maybe these brain regions that are important for addiction are also the same neural circuits that are important for responses to natural rewards including sex, food, and love. If the ability to become addicted helps animals bond to their mates, maybe that's why these neuro pathways are useful for the survival of the species—and why they persist even though addiction is harmful.

Pair bonding seems to form by condition learning in perhaps, these reward pathways. Among other things, the partner's smell, in the case of rodents, can become associated with the rewarding feelings of sex. Eventually, you want to be with the person who you're familiar with in these other ways.

Oxytocin has other effects that have been reported in animals and in humans. Oxytocin has a wide range of effects that we associate with pair bonding. For instance, it evokes feelings of contentment, reductions in anxiety, and feelings of calmness and security around a mate. Oxytocin levels are correlated with social bonding, increases in trust, and decreases in fear. All these things are things that we associate with pair bonding. These signals also turn up in several other contexts. One context is pregnancy and parenthood.

Let's follow these signaling molecules through pregnancy and parenthood. One major event is labor. When pregnant women are in labor, oxytocin is released in large amounts after distension of the cervix and vagina. Remember, I said that when these structures are stimulated oxytocin levels go up—well, there's no denying that labor is a very simulating experience. In childbirth, oxytocin triggers cervical dilation. In later stages of labor, oxytocin triggers contractions. Therefore, oxytocin is often given to women—and is called Pitocin—to induce delivery. A second time when oxytocin is secreted is after stimulation of the nipples. In this case, oxytocin secretion facilitates birth and also breastfeeding.

Recent studies have begun to investigate oxytocin's role in various behaviors. I've talked about several of them. In addition to pair bonding, there is also social recognition, orgasm, and maternal behaviors. Let's talk about those a little bit. Lactation. In lactation, these signaling molecules cause milk to drop. There is a reflex called "the letdown reflex" in which milk is let down into the subareolar sinuses. This is a place where milk can then be easily excreted through the nipple. Women can feel this; women can feel their milk drop. It is often the case that lactating women will report their milk dropping when they think about their babies. They feel a loving feeling or perhaps when they hear the baby crying. Women who are lactating will also report their milk dropping sometimes when they think about their life partners in a loving way. It appears that that same feeling of love can lead to the same psychological response, despite the fact that the functional role of that signal is different.

Here are some other examples of what I said before, that men and women are often quite similar in their brain circuitry. There are other similarities— now we're getting a little bit away from oxytocin, but some oxytocin related signaling. There are examples that happen post-birth. Obviously men don't get pregnant, but after the baby is born, there are parallels in men's and women's brain hormonal responses. One parallel between men and women is that sex hormone levels change. Estrogen levels go up in women; testosterone levels go down in men. Another way in which these signaling molecules may play a role in parenting is in the phenomenon of parental love. Mother's attachment to their children may involve some of the same neurocircuits as bonding with mate. I mentioned the milk dropping example. That's an example in which oxytocin may be involved.

Oxytocin is necessary for mother-infant bonding. For instance, if you take a rodent who's inexperienced and she's never had pups and you give her oxytocin, then instead of being aggressive towards the pups, which would be her normal tendency, she'll approach pups and try to care for them. Thus, it's possible to induce the feeling of parental nurturing in an inexperienced female rat. On the other hand, blocking oxytocin receptors during labor and delivery prevents rodent mothers from bonding with their pups. They are not very interested in taking care of their pups. Also, if you go and damage the reward areas that I mentioned before—the ventral tegmental area or the nucleus accumbens, both of which are associated with rewards in rodents—damage to these areas impairs the tendency of those rodents to care for their pups.

Brain changes during parenthood are not restricted to females. They also occur in men. One study that's very interesting has been done in marmosets. It's been done by colleagues of mine at Princeton, Genia Kozovoritskiy and Liz Gould. What they've done is they've studied changes in brain structure that are associated with parenting. In particular, they've studied increases in the shape and remodeling of dendrites. Remember that, earlier in the last lecture, I showed that estrogen can affect hippocampal dendrites. What they found is that in fact there's also a very interesting event that happens as a result of the act of parenting. Marmoset parents, when parenting for the first time, will show changes in their dendrites—this time not in the hippocampus, but in the prefrontal cortex. You can see spines sprouting in dendrites. This turns out to be true in male parents. It clearly is not associated with the act of pregnancy because it's in males. What's interesting here is that it's possible to see brain changes associated with the act of parenting.

Changes in human brains that are associated with parenting persist after birth in us and persist to about the end of the preschool period. There are hormonal changes that I mentioned before; these hormonal changes persist to the end of the preschool period. It seems to coincide with the period of time when we are most likely to be in physical contact with our children. It seems to coincide approximately with the time over which we handle babies a lot. With time, we handle them less and with time these hormonal levels revert back to where they were before the child was born. I've often wondered if this is why experienced parents so often reach for other people's babies. Perhaps they may want those feelings back again. You can see this in grandparents and parents. You can see this in people who know their way around a baby.

For the end, I want to now take one step further away and talk about phenomena such as trust and friendship. These are areas that are associated with the same signaling molecules. Let's think about, for instance, risk taking. If you've ever taken a stupid risk when you were in love and later wondered how you ever could have trusted that loser, then you might be interested to know that oxytocin seems to increase people's trust during social interactions—even with strangers. For example, oxytocin can be applied and get into the brain by intranasal application. For instance, if you do this, you can see changes in the way that a financial negotiation game turns out.

In one experiment, subjects were asked to play a game in which they could make money. The way it was done was this. You're an investor and you can make money by taking the risk of giving your money to a trustee. That trustee will then take your money and give it back to you, plus a bonus, and choose how much to give back to you. The trustee gets to decide how much you get back. If the trustee is trustworthy, both players benefit from your decision; otherwise, only the trustee benefits. Investors who were given a nasal spray of oxytocin were about twice as likely to give money to the trustee as those who were not given the drug. Thus, there's this change in trust behavior in response to oxytocin.

Interestingly, this effect was only seen when the trustee was a real person. If it was a computer who randomly decided how much money the investor would get, there was no difference. It appears that oxytocin is involved specifically in social interactions, not general risk taking. These results suggest that you might want to avoid making important financial decisions while under the influence of mind-altering substances like those released during orgasm.

What have we learned today about sexual behavior, love, and pair bonding? We've learned that sexual behavior leads back to the same place as sexual differentiation and sex differences—the hypothalamus. Sexual behavior and these structures are also connected with the stress response in ways that are important on an everyday basis for sexual behavior. I've talked about key brain signals for love and attachment—in particular, these two molecules, these two peptides, vasopressin and oxytocin. From voles, we've learned how important these molecules are, and their pathways, and their receptors are for pair bonding. These same signals may be important for parenting, bonding between mother and infant, trust, comfort, and perhaps even for friendship.

214

I'd like to close with a statement that was made once by the film director Woody Allen. He said, "My brain is my second favorite organ." Considering what we've learned today, I would submit to you that there's more in common between Mr. Allen's second favorite organ and his number one choice than he may have suspected.

Now that we've talked about sex differences and sex, what we'll do in the next lecture is we will turn to other functions that also seem mysterious. We're going to talk about explanations for them. We're going to talk about humor, math, and other curiosities of brain evolution.

Math and Other Evolutionary Curiosities
Lecture 32

> Why does humor exist and why [in] all these forms? ... It's not immediately clear how one could ever arrive at an adaptation-based explanation for these many forms of humor. After all, there's not really such a thing as a sarcastic rat or, for that matter, a sarcastic chimp.

A puzzle of human behavior is the existence of abilities in us with unknown survival value or with no clear antecedent among other animals—humor and math, for instance. Where did these capabilities come from, evolutionarily speaking? In general, the theory of natural selection posits that a selection advantage is necessary for a trait to become part of the heritage of a species.

Most behaviors have some antecedent in other animals: the fear response, the ability to detect and attract mates, the ability to pair bond, and the ability to avoid from danger. These behaviors have clear survival value and obviously measurable consequences. Two good examples of evolutionarily questionable capacities are humor and math. Why does humor exist, and why does it come in so many varieties? One can think of jokes, puns, slapstick, sarcasm, irony, and whimsy. Similarly, we have arithmetic, algebra, trigonometry, calculus, multivariate analysis, and the list goes on.

Humor may have its origins as a safety signal to others. Safety seems to be a feature of many forms of humor—slapstick, for example. It's a very primitive form of humor that is fundamentally based on the false appearance of injury. It's funny because there's a contradiction between the event and the actual hazard. Another possible explanation is that laughter is a signal to the social group that some event is of trivial consequence. This fits with the phenomenon that laughter is contagious in a group and with the idea of humor as a socially oriented safety signal.

More sophisticated humor involves cognition. A key component of a joke is a story that leads to a sudden flash of insight that happens in a moment when you have to reevaluate what was going on. Some patients with damage to the frontal lobes of the brain, in particular on the right side, don't get jokes at all, apparently because they have trouble with this reinterpretation stage of the process.

A harder question of evolutionary neuroscience is math. It appears that humans are unique in having the mental ability to do arithmetic. At its highest level, math is not seen in animals, but there are antecedents in other animals for certain rudimentary skills that go into math. The first is a sense of approximate number, or numerosity. If you look at a pile of objects, you can tell whether it has more or fewer than another pile. Another antecedent is an immediate sense of exact small numbers, or the ability to look at a number of objects and immediately know how many there are. This capability is called subitizing. These capacities have obvious selection

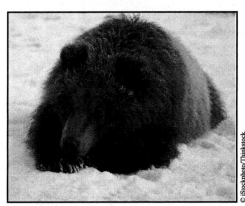

Some traits, such as a bear's fur coat, have clear functional advantages.

advantages. It's easy to imagine that they are useful in the everyday life of any animal. They are thought to be the foundation of our sense of math.

What we share with animals is numerosity and subitizing. What is added that allows us to do arithmetic and, perhaps, higher math? The unique human contribution comes with symbolic representations of number, which is a component of language—a sense of exact number with associated symbols. Arithmetic and other forms of math seem to consist of linking this symbolic representation of number with the approximate number sense. ∎

Questions to Consider

1. What is the role of exaptation in accounting for the origins of a specific trait?

2. In this lecture, two specific advanced mental capacities were discussed: humor and mathematics. Are there mental functions that seem to you to be out of reach of an evolutionary explanation?

Math and Other Evolutionary Curiosities
Lecture 32—Transcript

Welcome back. What I'd like to do in the coming lectures is to turn towards features of behavior that might be a little bit harder to account for, at least at first. What we're doing now is we're going to turn away from sex, sexual behavior, love, and pair bonding, whose functions are shared and recognizable across so many animal species. What I'd like to do in the coming lectures is talk about characteristics that seem uniquely human. What I'm going to do today is talk about evolutionary curiosities, things that seem unique to our species—but, perhaps, for which we could find a deeper evolutionary explanation. In particular, we'll be talking about things like humor and math.

A puzzle of human behavior is the existence of abilities in us with unknown survival value or with no clear antecedent among other animals. For instance, as I said, humor and math. One question we can ask is, what's within range of neuroscience and its associated disciplines—such as biology and psychology—for us to adequately explain or at least begin to explain? Some things have been easier to solve in detail. We've talked through this course about things such as primary sensory transduction for which explanations now exist at the cellular and molecular level. For more advanced functions, we've also talked about things like decision making, working memory, and fear—all kinds of things for which we can come up with biological explanations and some kind of coherent explanation.

In general, for all these functions, it's been possible to identify cells or brain regions that underlie these mechanisms. Today's topics are ones in which we will try do to the same thing, but there's an additional different challenge. The additional different challenge is to think of what are the levels of explanation that we need to account for—especially given that we are faced with the puzzle of where these capabilities arose in the first place. Where did these capabilities arise? What I mean by that is to ask the question, where did traits come from, evolutionary speaking? In general, the theory of natural selection poses that a selection advantage is necessary for a trait to become part of the species' heritage. In other words, if one individual has that trait, then it has some selection advantage in order for the trait to become part of its heritage.

We can see this over and over again with traits; we see the trait and we can see what its likely functional role is. Most behaviors, for instance, in the case of neurosciences, have some antecedent in other animals. We are animals. Thus, for instance, I'll pose examples such as the fear response, the ability to detect and attract mates, the ability to pair bond, and the ability to get away from danger. These are behaviors where we can see those traits in us and in other animals. Those are behaviors that have clear survival value and obviously measurable consequences. We would call these, generally speaking, "adaptive features." This is a major category of explanation in evolutionary theory—the idea that there's a feature or ability that arose with a clearly identifiable functional advantage.

I'll give you an example from biology—a bear's fur coat. When animals have fur coats such as bears, those fur coats have the clear advantage, functionally, of conferring warmth. Other features are harder to explain. For instance, birds have feathers and birds fly. However, predecessors to birds didn't fly. Feathers—which seem like a fairly complex feature—where did feathers come from? What could possibly have preceded feathers? Puzzles such as feathers on birds pose a much more interesting test of evolution as a conceptual framework. This is because, if evolution is to account as a logical framework for all of biology, it's necessary to look for causes of a phenomenon such as feathers. In the case of birds, the answer appears to be when you look at the fossil record and also when you look at pre-bird species, it appears to be the case that there are old feather-like structures that were originally useful as insulation for warmth, as the fur coat was. These feather-like features were then useful later for gliding and flight.

What I'd like to do is apply this general approach—adaptive and post-adaptive, which turns out to be called "exaptation"—to brain capacities, some of which at first seem difficult to explain. We have abilities that are of obvious survival value, as I've said—fear, memory, and stress responses. These are cases where abilities are of obvious survival value. But in other cases there are behavioral qualities, capacities that we have, that have no clear antecedent among other animals. In these cases, the question that I want to pose and partly answer—in this lecture—is how can we come up with an evolutionarily kind of explanation? Can we come up with a simpler behavior that appears earlier in the history of life and that appears in other animals, some simpler behavior that is in some ways matching, homologous, similar, to us so that we can see a possible candidate antecedent behavior?

The other type of explanation is one that we've covered over and over again in this course. That is biological mechanisms—mechanisms in terms of neurochemicals, neuronal circuits, and perhaps, in terms of development. In principle, biological mechanisms need to be consistent with the proposed evolutionary mechanism. Together, they form a coherent framework. For instance, in this lecture, we'll consider common brain structures that might be involved in one of these capacities in animals and in us.

What I'd like to focus on today are two capacities. I mentioned this at the beginning. I want to focus on these as two puzzles of evolutionary neurobiology. The two puzzles are humor and math. We'll consider both of them at turn, humor being seemingly more of an emotional category of behavior, and math more of a cognitive category.

Let's think about humor. Humor comes in many varieties—jokes, puns, slapstick, sarcasm, and irony. Humor is multifaceted. Why does humor exist and why all these forms? One can think of sarcasm, irony, and whimsy. It's not immediately clear how one could ever arrive at an adaptation-based explanation for these many forms of humor. After all, there's not really such a thing as a sarcastic rat or, for that matter, a sarcastic chimp.

A second example I want to talk about is a more cognitively oriented example—math. Again, this is a case where we're far from animals. In this case, we are seemingly very far from other animals. Let's just think about a few different forms of math. We have arithmetic, algebra, higher forms of math, trigonometry, calculus, multivariate calculus, probability, topology, and the list goes on. Math comes in many forms. Again, these are functions that appear to be very far from other animals. If we look at these, seemingly they don't seem very related to what animals in general can do. But it turns out that more thought and closer examination reveals at least the possibility of a natural explanation based on what other animals are capable of doing.

Let's consider humor. What I propose to do now is to start analyzing humor in scientific terms. At this point, I feel compelled to quote the writer E.B. White who said that "humor can be dissected as a frog can, but the thing dies in the process and the innards are discouraging to any but the pure scientific mind." Luckily, you have a pure scientific mind in your presence here and so I'm going to start dissecting humor.

Humor is hard to define, but we know it when we see it. We know what humor is when we hear a joke or when we see something funny happen. But, I want to pose to you the core problem—where did humor come from? I'll pose this to you as a possible framework for the origins of humor. Humor may have its origins as a safety signal to others. Imagine you're walking in a dark part of your house. Imagine it's getting dark, you're alone, it's a little bit scary, and then you hear something fall. Is it an intruder? Then you look and it's the cat. Ha ha, it's the cat. That would be an example of a safety signal. Safety then seems to be a feature of many forms of humor.

In addition, humor also seems to be a source of pleasure. Humor makes people feel good. It appears to do so by activating the brain reward areas that respond to other pleasures like food and sex. This can be seen in brain scanning experiments involving humor. For instance, when pleasures are coupled with surprise, a sense of pleasure could even trigger a smile or laughter. What's going on here? Well, let's think about what's going on.

First, let's try to go back, the way that one would go back on the evolutionary tree and go look at simpler and simpler forms of humor. Certainly jokes can be complex and subtle. But, imagine a very early form of humor—slapstick. It's a very primitive form of humor. It's considered a lower form of humor and perhaps it might be easier to explain. Slapstick is fundamentally based on the false appearance of injury. Think about the elements; it's got a pratfall, so you fall or you appear to fall, mock violence, and then the person gets up. You can see mock violence followed by the appearance of no injury. Imagine *The Three Stooges,* where you put the fingers in the eyes and the other guy goes "na, na, na."

That kind of thing is slapstick. It's funny because there's a contradiction between the event and the actual hazard where you are poking the guy in the eyes and then the guy is not actually injured. This is because, of course, actual injury is not funny. If you actually took a person and went like that into the eyes, that would not be funny. Most people do not find that kind of thing, actual injury, to be funny. There's an exception which is sociopaths. Sociopaths often find actual injury to be funny, although, even in these cases, these people still do not think it's funny when they are injured. Thus, slapstick gives a little bit of insight into where humor might come from.

Let's think about physical expressions of emotion. The physical expressions of emotion were interesting to Darwin and to many investigators afterward. We talked about this previously when talking about emotions. Let's think about major emotional expressions of humor. Let's think about smiles. The neurologist V.S. Ramachandran has written about smiles as possibly grimaces that don't make it all the way. He points out that, when a primate encounters another primate, the first thing the primate does is to make a threat, to bare the canines. But, it turns out, if the other individual is kin, the primate will stop halfway. It becomes a smile where partially bared canines, partially exposed teeth, constitute a smile. So, a smile might be a threat gesture that doesn't make it all the way. It's a threat gesture that gets halfway to being a threat and then stops. That's a possible explanation for what a smile is and where smiling came from.

Another example is laughter. Laughter is this funny expulsion repeatedly of air and the sound that goes with it. One possibility for laughter is that it's an ancestral signal for a situation that seemed dangerous but is actually safe. That is a possible explanation for laughter. If we go back to pre-scientific investigations of laughter, Freud thought that perhaps laugher was discharging pent-up tension. The idea is that there's tension inside you and then the tension is discharged. He had sort of a hydraulic explanation for laughter. I'm not sure how one would interpret that other than the fact that what appears to be going on there is a re-description of the phenomena itself. Another possible explanation is that laughter is a signal to your social group that some event is of trivial consequence. You thought it was dangerous, but it turns out to be safe.

This fits with the phenomenon that laughter is contagious in a group. If one person starts laughing, then other people will laugh as well. Certainly, that seems to fit with the idea of laughter as a socially oriented safety signal. It certainly accounts for slapstick humor. Something that was dangerous turns out not to be dangerous.

Let's now move on to more sophisticated aspects of humor. Let's move on from slapstick to things such as jokes. I want to pose the general question, how does your brain know that a joke is funny? Let's think about jokes. A key component of a joke is a story that leads to a sudden flash of insight. That sudden flash of insight happens in a moment when you have to reevaluate what was going on. You were told a story—you know, a duck walks into a bar or whatever it might be—and then something happens and you have to reevaluate what was going on. Neurological patients often have trouble with jokes. Some patients with damage to the frontal lobes of the brain, in particular on the right side, don't get jokes at all. This appears to be because they have trouble with this reinterpretation stage of the process. For instance, if you take one of these patients and give him or her a joke with the choice of punch lines, that person cannot tell which punch line would be funny.

Conversely, it is possible to trigger feelings of amusement. It's possible to trigger feelings of amusement in some of these same brain regions. For instance, laughter or amused feelings have been evoked in epileptic patients when you put in probes to look for the epileptic region. You can actually stimulate the prefrontal cortex or the lower part of the temporal cortex. You can see that these regions, when activated, lead to feelings of something funny happening. Functional imaging studies—if you take a person and put that person in the scanner—show that the orbital and medial prefrontal cortex are active when people get a joke. Humor includes both emotional and cognitive components. It makes sense that these prefrontal regions, which integrate those two functions, might be involved in the detection of humor.

Multiple types of humor, when tested in the scanner, activate areas that respond to emotional stimuli as well. I'll list a few of them and these will be familiar to you, at least some of them will be, from our discussions of emotion. Brain regions that are activated during humor include the amygdala, the midbrain, the anterior cingulate cortex, and the insular cortex. These are, I hope, familiar to you—especially these last two regions, the anterior cingulate and the insula. These two regions are also active in situations of uncertainty and incongruity. They might conceivably participate in the reinterpretation stage of getting a joke. Indeed, the funnier a person thinks the joke is, the more active these areas are; and the more active the reward regions of the brain are. Recall that I talked before, when I talked about emotion, about the anterior cingulate. I said that the anterior cingulate was involved in the phenomenon of reappraisal when we reevaluate the emotional impact of an experience. Humor often has an element of that. From slapstick to irony to sarcasm, reevaluation is quite frequent in those forms of humor.

Now I've covered a somewhat more complex form of humor. This opens up the way for other kinds of humor. Think about fairly advanced and less often appreciated forms of humor. Think of puns, irony, and sarcasm. These are so-called "higher forms of humor" and they seem to also do the same thing. They also seem to build upon a basic sense of incongruity or of reevaluation. It could be that these higher forms have the advantage, for instance, it might be they have the advantage of helping you link up unrelated ideas. This is because, after all, those are forms of humor that involve connecting up unrelated ideas.

It's less obvious that there's strong survival value to having those forms of a sense of humor. After all, a sense of humor varies among people just as cognitive ability varies among people. For example, it's observed commonly—you know this in your everyday life—that some persons only understand slapstick and mock cruelty, or perhaps even not-so-mock cruelty. Those are the things that are most funny to some people. I have to say that I generally regard such a sense of humor as being cognitively unsophisticated, but nonetheless, that is a form of a sense of humor.

Humor also has medical benefits. Humor's rewards go beyond simply feeling good. For instance, being talented at making other people laugh can improve all kinds of social interactions. It can help you find a mate and it can help you communicate your ideas more effectively. It's been observed, in the literature, that humor also reduces the effects of stress on the heart, immune system, and hormones. Given what I've told you about stress, the immune system, and hormonal signaling, this perhaps should not be surprising since I've talked about emotional systems that are connected to those systems of signaling. If you're the kind of person who tends to be amused by things that other people don't find funny, then you may in fact get the last laugh.

Let's tackle what seems to be a harder one, a harder question of evolutionary neuroscience. That one is math. Math seems to be a pretty advanced capacity. It appears that we are unique in having the mental ability to do arithmetic. It appears that we can't study math, per se, in other animals. At one point, it was thought that was the case. There was a famous case of a horse named Hans. Hans was able to clop out answers to arithmetic problems correctly. His master, a man named Wilhelm Von Osten, was often in the habit of showing him off and took him on exhibitions. It emerged that clever Hans turned out to be basically clopping his foot until Wilhelm Von Osten moved his body. He basically used body language to communicate with Hans. Even subconsciously, it was possible for Hans, without verbal communication, to pick up unintended signals from human masters to know when to stop clopping. At its highest level, math is not really seen in animals. However, even though the clever Hans case mainly shows the difficulty of studying such things, there are antecedents in other animals for certain rudimentary skills that go into math. These antecedent skills are ones that we also have. I'll provide the two main ones.

The first antecedent is a sense of approximate number, the sense of numerosity. If you look at a pile of marbles or other objects, you can tell whether it has more objects or fewer objects than another one. That's one sense that we share with animals. Even children and infants have a sense of numerosity. Another sense is an immediate sense of exact small numbers. This is a sense that can work up to about seven objects. This is a sense in which you can just look at a number of objects and immediately see whether there are two, three, four, or whatever number of objects. This capability is called "subitizing" and it comes from a Latin word that means sudden. What it refers to is the idea that you can suddenly, immediately, tell just how many objects there are in front of you. Subitizing along with numerosity are two fundamental skills than one can look at, two capabilities that we can look at. We can also see them, as I said, in other animals.

These capacities have obvious selection advantages. I talked before about adaptation and selection advantages. It is possible to easily imagine what these are good for. You can use them to know which food source is more abundant. You can use them to figure out which situation is more dangerous. If you have two possible enemies versus three possible enemies, the three are more dangerous than the two. It's easy to imagine that these capabilities are useful in the everyday life of any animal.

These two systems—approximate number numerosity, and small exact numbers, subitizing—are found early in life and even found in other animals. They are thought to be the foundation of our sense of math. We can see these, for instance, in chimpanzees. For instance, a chimpanzee will spontaneously select between options of trays. A chimpanzee will spontaneously pick trays that have more chocolate bits than ones that have fewer chocolate bits. What this demonstrates is that chimps have some ability to compare approximate numerosities. They can even do so with multiple trays. Thus, they have to do some form of rudimentary addition where, if they have multiple trays, they can pick a pair of trays with more bits of chocolate than other trays. They can do that as well. It's possible to see this sense of general numerosity in other animals. It's possible to see it not only in chimps, but you can even see it in mice, dogs, and even pigeons. That's an example of numerosity in other animals.

Another example of what you can see in other animals is a sense of exact number. For instance, early in development, you can find this in infants and children. Recall I talked about infants having cognitive capabilities as early as the age of three months. Infants are good at telling the exact number of objects. If you have an object come up—say a little mouse doll or something like that—you put the object in front of the infant. You put up a barrier. Then, you add another object of the same type that goes behind the barrier. You then take away the barrier. You know that there are two objects behind the barrier. The infants are surprised if there's only one. They'll look longer if they see only one object versus two. Therefore, it's possible to track this number sense in infants.

It's also possible to track whether infants care about other things as well. Infants care much more about the number of objects than the identity of the objects. For instance, infants are not terribly surprised if a duck goes behind the barrier and then a truck comes out, or if a truck goes in and a duck comes out. Infants don't care so much about the appearance of the object, but they do care about the number. In other words, infants can subitize.

Infants can also track approximate numbering. Again, you can see this fairly early; you can see this in six-month-old infants. In six-month-old infants, you can show them numbers of dots. You can show them one number of dots and then another dot pattern and another dot pattern. If the number of dots suddenly changes, infants will look longer. Again, this demonstrates that they're able to tell that something's a little bit more or less. Roughly speaking, six-month-olds can tell when one group is twice as large or half as large as another. The ratio that six-month-olds can distinguish is about 2 to 1.

This capacity gets better with age and ultimately gets to about a ratio of 7 to 8 in adults. We can tell when something is changed by about one-seventh or one-eighth. That's a change that we are able to detect. By the way, it's interesting that this approximate number sense is also associated with better arithmetic abilities as children get older. For instance, having a good number sense early in life is correlated with having better arithmetic abilities as children get older. Among other things, that supports the idea that these two senses—numerosity and subitizing—might be important in forming basic abilities for math and arithmetic. It suggests even the possibility—and this is a speculative possibility—that you could train that numerosity sense and perhaps improve arithmetic.

In other words, if you're trying to teach a small child, exact arithmetic might not be the only thing that could be trained. One can imagine that children could be taught to do approximate number problems to eventually improve their arithmetic skills. This hasn't been tested adequately, but it's certainly an intriguing possibility for ways that we could work with children to help them be better at math.

I hope I've persuaded you that there is some possible evolutionary reason, some possible antecedents, for our sense of arithmetic and math in other animals and babies. Now what I'd like to do is just spend a little bit of time talking about how number is represented in the brain. This has been investigated at the level of brain scanning. In particular, it has been possible to put a person in the brain scanner and then look at patterns of brain activity. It has also been possible to look at people with brain damage and see whether they're able to process language, but not math, or perhaps they can still do math, but not process language. In particular, there are cases of acalculia in which people are verbal and can have perfectly good conversations, but can't calculate. There's even a converse disorder in which people, when asked to write, just scribble. They make meaningless scribbles. But, when it comes time to do math problems, they can do perfectly good math problems. They can do multiplication. They can do fairly sophisticated things. These demonstrate that there's something about arithmetic ability that is separated from other abilities such as language. If we look at these kinds of evidence from brain scanning data and also from brain lesion data, it appears that numerical information is represented in regions of the prefrontal and posterior parietal lobes. In particular, there's this one part of the brain that seems to be very important for semantic number content, for remembering things like the number 27, or whatever it might be. That particular region is a groove, a sulcus—which is what a groove is in the brain—called "the intraparietal sulcus." The intraparietal sulcus appears to be a key location where this semantic number content is represented.

It also appears to be the case—when we study people both by testing them and also by looking in these brain regions—that there is a mental number line. This mental number line seems to be involved in this sense of numerosity, which is also known as "cardinality." It's that sense of approximate number. For instance, if I were to ask you what's larger, eight or three, most subjects can answer that fairly quickly. But, people have more difficulty and take a little bit longer when comparing eight and three than if they're asked to compare eight with seven. If I say which is larger, eight or seven, despite the fact that that's not a hard problem, it takes noticeably longer, measurably longer, to tell eight from seven than from three, and similarly, four from three. In fact, it's also harder to tell eight from seven than it is to tell four from three. What this seems to indicate is the possibility of closer numbers are actually closer to one another in mental space. It's as if numbers are represented in the brain in some kind of mental number line. We're moving things or manipulating these numbers as if they're close or far from one another in mental space.

There's a very interesting finding that has come out in the last few years which is it has started to come out that there are brain regions that don't seem to be involved in these fundamental functions, but they do seem to be involved in arithmetic. They seem to have other functions that have older significance and significance in other body functions. There's a very particular case I wanted to tell you about which is this: It turns out that brain regions that play a role for moving the eyes are also activated when we do mental arithmetic, for instance, when we do addition and subtraction problems. This is true even when the eyes are not observed to move. So these are brain regions that were originally studied because they seem to be involved in eye movements and people have been interested in them for a long time. When looking at these, investigators looked at this with the hope of finding something that might be correlated with more complex mental manipulation such as arithmetic. It's possible when people looked for brain regions that were involved in addition and subtraction, it's possible to see fMRI signatures of addition and subtraction, and in particular it's possible to watch a person doing addition and subtraction problems over and over and over again. And if you watch enough of them, it takes a lot, you have to watch many, many instances of this, you can then use that to build a model for what happens in that person's brain when he or she adds or subtracts. Then you can take that and look at another case and take a guess as to whether that person is adding or subtracting. It turns out that your guess is going to be much better than chance. It's going to be better than chance and you can tell whether the person is adding or subtracting by looking at brain regions that are involved in eye movement.

Let's get back to this adaptation/exaptation hypothesis. This observation suggests that these structures that control eye movement probably originally arose to perform a necessary function in non-human animals, the movement of the eyes which is after all, universal, and they were co-opted for other uses. This co-opting then for manipulating numbers by mentally looking to figure out whether something is a larger or smaller number, or whatever it is that one does in mental arithmetic. This co-opting might be a mechanism by which these brain regions were then recruited into service for something very different. As I mentioned before, I've used the word "exaptation." Exaptation is a term for an existing feature that gets co-opted for use in a new function.

There's very famous essay by the evolutionary biologist the late Stephen J. Gould about exaptation and the essay is called, "The Spandrels of St. Marco." It's about St. Mark's Cathedral in Venice in which, when you have a dome and then you have arches, you have these upside-down triangular regions in which paintings have been put. What he pointed out was that those triangle regions were not for the paintings. What happened was that, in fact, when architects designed the cathedral they had these triangular spaces and they needed to put something there. So that's an example of exaptation where there's a triangle and then it was called into use.

Let's now start connecting this together a little bit. Before, I talked about what we shared with animals, numerosity, and subitizing. What is it that's added that allows us to do arithmetic and perhaps higher math? Well, the unique human contribution comes with symbolic representations of number. This is a component of language. So what we're talking about now is a sense of exact number with symbols associated. Arithmetic and other forms of math seem to consist of linking this symbolic representation of number with the approximate number sense. Of course this leaves the remaining puzzle, the remaining puzzle is a deep one which is, where do symbols and language come from? Now it has become merged with another fundamental question which is, where does language come from? Of course language is a form of representing information in shorthand, clearly useful in a social animal like us. I have to say at this point the trail gets a little bit fuzzier. I have to say that the neural basis of language is not terribly well understood, but a lot of interesting work has been done by psychologists and by linguists. So to understand language better, one could look in the writings of influential linguists such as Noam Chomsky at MIT who has come up with a theory of generative grammar in which rules are used to construct utterances. Those rules then get put together in order to generate language. Another place to look for interesting insights on this is popular writings by Steven Pinker who has written about language.

So what have we learned today? Well, what I hope you've gotten out of this is that the comparative method of comparing animals with one another, or even looking at different stages of development, that the comparative method is a powerful one to understand where behaviors may have come from. I have given two examples, humor and math, to show that even higher functions often have antecedents when you look in other animals. I want to close with a general observation. You will often find press accounts that are based in evolutionary psychology. I have just given you, in fact, two possible explanations based on evolution. These claims are often hard to evaluate. One way to evaluate those claims is to look at other animals to see if the same principle holds. Another way to do it is to look in terms of biological mechanism and to start asking if at a level of neural circuitry whether the principle makes sense at the level of the actual mechanisms that are used to generate these behaviors. The general principle then from an evolutionary sense is that what appears to be the case is that complex functions are often built on simpler prior functions. I want to leave you with that, with the principle of exaptation, the spandrel hypothesis.

In the next lecture what we'll do is we'll go onto other forms of fairly complex, somewhat mysterious, phenomenon. In the next lecture we'll cover consciousness and free will.

Consciousness and Free Will
Lecture 33

What is it in the brain that produces the quality of "cold" or "blue"? ... What it is in the brain that produces this quality in the sense of what I feel, or perhaps what I imagine that you might feel? This seemingly simple question perplexes scientists partly because it defines the question in terms of unmeasurable aspects of experience.

The idea of **consciousness** contains two components: One is the state of being awake and able to respond to our environment, and the second is awareness of experience or thought. The fundamental concept for neuroscience in regard to consciousness is that a physical process of neural activity is responsible for the subjective phenomenon of awareness. This idea seems impossible; thus, there is some kind of fundamental gap to be bridged between the physical and the subjective. One approach is to seek a neural correlate of consciousness, a specific pattern of activity that correlates with a particular conscious experience.

Another way to think about consciousness is that it seems to have essential components. One is attention; another seems to be working memory, in the sense that when we are consciously aware, we can remember what happened before—a stream of consciousness. This combination seems to be a good provisional way to think about conscious awareness.

Conscious awareness may be overrated as a guide of behavior.

Conscious awareness may be overrated as a guide of behavior. For instance, our perception of the world is continuous, despite blinking or moving the eyes. We are able to discard that information because, if we perceived all that information, we would be distracted. The clear implication is that perception, while continuous, is in some sense a filtered version of what happens when we receive visual information from the world. The phenomenon of "blind sight," the ability of people with visual impairment to carry on activities of daily living, indicates that there are ways in which conscious awareness is unnecessary for navigating through the world.

The question of free will presents an apparent paradox to anyone interested in the philosophy of the brain. The physical model of how the brain works is that our experience, desires, thoughts, emotions, and reactions seem to be generated by the brain's physical activity. The implication is that physical and chemical laws govern all thoughts and actions: You are your brain. Yet every day, you make choices and act upon the world around you. How can these facts be reconciled?

The practical implications of what we know about brain function are perhaps less complicated than the philosophical contemplation of free will. A practical definition of free will is based on predictability. But even single synapses are unpredictable, so predicting the details of what a whole brain will do is impossible. From a practical standpoint, that's a definition of freedom and, perhaps, of free will.

In answer to the question of whether we should change the brain to influence behavior, the Dalai Lama said that such a treatment would have saved him time spent in meditation, freeing him up to do more good works. But he also said that such a treatment would be acceptable only if it left one's critical faculties intact.

This caveat raises the point of moral responsibility for our actions. For instance, is it possible to separate our actions from our capacity for moral reasoning? From the standpoint of everyday life, conceptual difficulties with the question of free will are resolved in a practical sense with the idea that you are responsible for all your actions. You are your brain and your brain is responsible for your actions. ■

Important Term

consciousness: The awareness of oneself and the world in a subjective sense.

1. What does Benjamin Libet's experiment tell us about whether we have free will?

2. What is the role of punishment in our society for criminal actions? Do you think this role—or even punishment itself—may change in the future?

Consciousness and Free Will
Lecture 33—Transcript

Welcome back. In the last lecture we talked about humor, math, other phenomena that seem like evolutionary curiosities, until you look at them a little bit more closely. Now what I'd like to do in the coming lectures is to talk about some rather big ideas. In this lecture what I'm going to do is I'm going to cover a fairly big idea and it's one of the original reasons why I became a neuroscientist in the first place, and this problem is the problem of consciousness and free will. This is something that interested me for a long time from when I was a child.

For those of us neuroscientists who were drawn in for philosophical reasons, one of the tyrannies of picking our field is that we originally came into the field wanting to understand some very fundamental issues of existence. As I said, the existence of free will, the self, that kind of thing. That's as opposed to other areas of biologies. So, for example, consider cell biology. Cell biologists are often drawn into their field by very interesting puzzles, how particular parts of cells work, how some kind of trafficking, say inside cells or between cells takes place, and then they work on those puzzles and then they get to solve them.

Neuroscientists who come in for philosophical reasons often typically end up working on more tractable problems, and these problems usually lack the original philosophical romance, with some exceptions. What that means is that in some respects, neuroscientists end up in the same boat as everyone else in terms of having a sense of who we are. One thing that I should say though is that it is now possible for neuroscience to show some ways that we can start thinking about problems of identity a little bit more concretely. So what I'd like to do today is take you through how one could start experimenting with phenomena such as consciousness or such as the question of free will.

Let's consider consciousness. When we use the word "consciousness" as a colloquial term, and if you start looking at it more closely and asking what is consciousness, it's possible to identify two different aspects of consciousness. And when we use that word sometimes we mean one, sometimes we mean the other. Let's consider the two aspects of consciousness. So one aspect is in some sense the easy definition of consciousness, and that's the state of being conscious, and that's as opposed to being unconsciousness. So, for example, when we're awake we're conscious. When we are awake we are able to respond to our environments, we can move around, and this state of consciousness is something that does not happen, for instance, when we're asleep. The state of consciousness, of being conscious, depends on parts of the nerve system called the "ascending reticular activating system." These are columns of neurons in the brain stem whose activity is high when we're awake and low when we are not awake. So that sense of consciousness is one definition of consciousness.

There's a second definition. As opposed to being conscious there's the question of being conscious of X, and so for instance if I see a green apple and I think to myself there's a green apple in front of me, then I am conscious of that green apple. So that's a second sense of consciousness, that I am paying attention to something and I can see that object in front of me. This second sense of consciousness is a particular mental state that people have been very interested in and has started to be investigated in the last few decades.

So one could start posing it first as a philosophical question and then perhaps turn it into a neuro-scientific question. I would pose the question as, what is it in the brain that produces the quality of cold or blue? So for instance, if I see blue or if you feel cold, what it is in the brain that produces this quality in the sense of what I feel or perhaps what I imagine that you might feel?

This seemingly simple question perplexes scientist because it defines the question partly because it defines the question in terms of unmeasurable aspects of experience. When philosophers think about the mind and think about how the brain might produce mind, philosophers call these immeasurable aspects of experience "qualia." So a fundamental question then is, how does the brain produce qualia? Here's the fundamental concept. The fundamental concept that permeates neuroscience in regards to the question of consciousness is that a physical process, the physical process of neural activity, this thing that we've been talking about, neurons firing, synapses releasing neurotransmitters, biochemical processes taking place in neurons and perhaps glia, these physical processes in principle are responsible for the subjective phenomenon of awareness. Let's think about that for a moment.

There's a physical process that leads to the idea that I'm here, and I'm looking at you, and I'm talking about neuroscience. So there's that disjunct between the physical process and the subjective phenomenon of awareness. This idea seems very hard to grasp and seems impossible in some ways to some philosophers. There is some kind of fundamental gap that needs to be bridged there between the physical and the subjective.

One way that a neuroscientist could address this question is to look for a physical phenomenon that is there when we are consciously aware. So the second kind of consciousness I talked about. In particular, one thing that we can look for is a neural correlate. In every other aspect of things that I've talked about in this course I've talked about brain activity that seems to correlate with a particular phenomenon such as smelling a smell or perhaps seeing a sunset or what have you. So now what we're talking about here is we're asking the question, can we find a neural correlate of consciousness, a specific pattern of activity that correlates with a particular conscious experience? So, if neuroscientists could define activity that occurs only when you notice a stimulus and never at any other time, then it could be legitimately claimed that we're studying brain activity that's related to conscious awareness. This is a way to possibly explain qualia, at least to find a physical phenomenon that corresponds to this word that I've given you, this philosophical word "qualia."

We can also think about consciousness in terms of its components, and so there's another way to think about consciousness, conscious awareness. That's that consciousness seems to have essential components. One essential component is attention, paying attention to a person or a thing or some event that's happening in your environment. Attention is one essential component of consciousness. Another component of consciousness seems to be working memory in the sense that when we are consciously aware we can remember what happened before. So if I walk across the campus at my university and I'm aware of what's going on around me, I can see what's happening, and I'm also generally aware of what happened immediately beforehand. There's this stream of consciousness, this stream of awareness that I have. It appears that consciousness is this stream of continuous experience in which we are continuously aware of events and we can remember them into the immediate past. So this combination of attention and working memory seems to be a good provisional way to think about what conscious awareness is.

It's possible to start asking questions like, okay, well, let's say that attention and working memory, let's say that this is what conscious awareness is. Well, let's ask a simple question. How much information is available to conscious awareness? The answer is not that much. So it turns out that a lot of brain activity does not meet these criteria of being accessible to conscious awareness. Take, for example, the visual system. We've talked about the visual system a lot because we're such visual animals. The primary visual cortex, the first place after the thalamus that visual information stops in the cortex, the primary visual cortex contains information about which eye is receiving a piece of information. So for instance if I'm shown one piece of information to my left eye, the other to my right eye, the visual cortex contains information about which eye received the information. But this is information that is not available to my conscious awareness. This is an example of the attentional spotlight, the idea that there are things that I'm aware of, that I can specifically call up to my awareness and others that I can't.

Here's an example of the converse of the attentional spotlight, attentional blindness. So here's an experiment in attentional blindness. If subjects are presented with two sets of pictures in quick succession, one, two, one, two, one, two, and they are asked to detect some feature that's in the first set of pictures, so if I show you one, two, one, two, and I ask you to look at something that's in one, then you concentrate on the first set of pictures. It turns out that concentrating on the first set of pictures makes it hard to detect a particular feature in the second set. This phenomenon of not being able to see things consciously in the second set is known as "attentional blindness."

That's the phenomenon of attentional blindness. In the face of that, despite that, there are brain regions that are activated every time that the second stimulus is presented, whether subjects report perceiving the stimulus or not. So for example, let's get back to the primary visual cortex. The second sets of images in one, two, one, two, one, two, the two images still generate activity in the primary visual cortex. So as a result, that's another piece of evidence that the primary visual cortex seems to not participate in what we call the "attentional spotlight."

In contrast, let's look at other cortical regions. There are other brain regions that are activated only on the repetitions when subjects report that they can see the second stimulus. So sometimes in this experiment subjects are able to see the second stimulus, when they're asked to or on other occasions. In these occasions it turns out that there is sometimes brain activity in other parts of the brain that are activated, and those are a neural correlate of the awareness of the second stimulus.

What this experiment shows is that visual stimuli can activate a surprisingly large number of brain regions, the primary visual cortex, including many steps leading up to the primary visual cortex. So visual stimuli can activate many brain regions without entering into conscious awareness, as if conscious awareness is like a spotlight. So when we take all the information that comes into us, all the information that comes through all our senses, there's a spotlight that focuses on specific stimuli and ignores others. That's the attentional spotlight.

It is possible to argue that conscious awareness, however vaunted by philosophers, it may be that conscious awareness is in fact, in some sense, overrated as a guide of behavior. For instance, vision can tell us about the importance or unimportance of conscious awareness. Looking at how we process vision can teach us something about how important it is to be consciously aware. I'll pose you a few examples from everyday life. For example, what happens when you blink your eyes? When you blink your eyes, your perception of the world is continuous. When you move your eyes from one place to another, despite the fact that the image of the world moves quite radically on your retinas, your perception of the world is continuous. So there appears to be something that happens when you blink or when you move your eyes, in which you are able to, in some sense, blank out what it is that you're looking at and not use that information. After all if you think about it, if you perceived all that information when you move your eyes or blink, you would be in fact very distracted. You'd constantly have the world cutting out for fractions of a second, or perhaps the world would suddenly swing around. So clearly what this seems to imply is that your perception, while continuous, is in some sense a filtered version of what happens when you receive visual information from the world.

Here's another example, recall the phenomena of blind sight. Recall that blind sight is a phenomenon in which people can respond to the visual world, can do things like mail a letter or perhaps catch a ball, despite the fact that they have damage to their visual cortex, so that's blind sight. Blind sight is a demonstration of the fact that conscious awareness only extends to a fraction of incoming stimuli. There's other information that we are not aware of consciously that is available for our brain's use. In this condition of blind sight, people can't report any details consciously of the world around them and for most purposes they're partially blind. What this means then is that there are cutouts in our conscious awareness. There are ways in which our conscious awareness is unnecessary for navigating through the world.

Here's another example of the overratedness of conscious awareness. Recall a gambling task that I described in a previous lecture, a gambling task in which one deck is stacked against the player and the player starts getting a sense that, in fact, it's time to start picking from another deck. This is called the "Iowa Gambling Task." This Iowa Gambling Task, developed at the University of Iowa, shows that there's information that's available to us without our being aware of it. It can often be quite complex, in this case this gap between hunch and recognition is something that can be measured in this pretend gambling game. What happens in this game is that people are given decks to draw from, recall, and they start avoiding one deck and they start picking from another one. They do this without being consciously aware of what's going on. This is an example of a task in which the people playing the game form a sense of what to do, change their behavior, and yet don't become consciously aware of what's going on until much later.

These two examples, visual awareness and the Iowa Gambling Task, show us that conscious awareness then is something that is not really necessary for navigating in a smooth way through the world. So consciousnesses in short, as I said, might be overrated.

Now let's turn to the other concept that I had mentioned in the beginning of this lecture, the other concept being the concept of free will. The question of free will presents an apparent paradox to anyone interested in the philosophy of how the brain works. I mentioned before this physical model of how the brain works. I said, on the one hand, your everyday experience, your desires, thoughts, emotions, and reactions, all seem to be generated by the physical activity of your brain. Experimental evidence supports that and that's the fundamental framework of neuroscience. Yet it's also true that the neurons and glia of your brain generate chemical changes leading to electrical impulses and cell-to-cell communication. So the implication then is that physical and chemical laws govern all your thoughts and actions. This proposition is at the core of the field of neuroscience. To put it briefly, you are your brain, yet every day you make choices and act upon the world around you. So how can these facts be reconciled? You are the result of physical forces and you seem to think that you have free will. How does the existence of these hidden processes, these physical processes, fit with the concept of free will? So let's think about free will.

I told you about conscious awareness. I told you about the fact that it perhaps might be a little bit overrated. Now let's think about a practical example of free will. So imagine you're walking down the street, you're walking down the street and it's a rainy day and there's a puddle in front of you. You step around the puddle and you're around the puddle. If you think about what you just did there, you didn't think about that until you were past the puddle. So you probably didn't say, I'm thinking about the puddle, there's the puddle, I'm going to step around the puddle, I go around it. No, what you probably did is you probably stepped around it and maybe halfway once you're past the puddle you said, oh puddle. So assuming that your feet end up dry at the end of this thought experiment, there's something about your free will that is coming along seemingly for the ride.

It's possible to capture this sense of free will or the timing of when apparently free will takes place, in a classic experiment that's very famous both among neuroscientists and also among non-neuroscientists. It's an experiment done by the late Benjamin Libet. Libet designed an experiment that shows that lack of awareness extends to our own actions. What he and his collaborators did in the 1980s was ask people to do a very simple experiment.

The experiment goes like this. You sit in a room and you have a measurement apparatus attached to you to measure when you tap your finger to measure muscle contraction, and there's a clock with a sweep hand, a very fast moving second hand. You're asked to do this, tap your finger a time of your own choosing, and note the time of your decision by looking at the clock with a sweep hand. So you look at the sweep hand and say, okay well, I made my decision to tap my finger at this particular time on the clock. In this experiment it's possible to measure different events. It's possible to measure brain activity in the form of EEG. It's possible to measure when you think that you made your decision to tap your finger, and it's possible to measure the tap of the finger itself. This is the result that Libet and his collaborators got.

They found that brain regions responsible for triggering movements started generating activity about half a second before any movement was made. So there's this electrical signal in the EEG called a "readiness potential," and this readiness potential started generating activity about half a second before the movement was made. But if you look at what the subject said as being the moment of awareness of their decision, they reported awareness of their decision a few tenths of a second later, right before the movement begin.

So to summarize, this is the order of events that they saw. They saw preparatory activity in the form of this readiness potential, then they saw reported self-awareness of the decision by the subject, and finally they saw movement. The fact that the readiness potential precedes the awareness or the subjective sense of making a decision seems to contradict our everyday idea of free will. The idea being that the conscious decision to take action, an event that we associate with free will, only comes after the stirrings of the action have already been initiated in the brain. So it appears to be the case that there's a neural commitment to decision before we become aware of making the decision.

There's an exception to this experiment in the Libet experiment. The exception is if those subjects were sometimes asked to stop a movement that was already initiated. There was some signal that told them to stop it, and in some sense they still had a veto right until the last moment, a veto that one could call "free won't." There has been a problem brought up with this experiment since it was originally done. The problem being that these subjects only had one choice, and so you tap or don't tap and it was basically go, don't go. So the question is well, does that preparatory readiness potential really reflect commitment to a choice, or is it just some kind of general readiness to do something? Could a better experiment be done? There has been another experiment that's better that's been done in which subjects have two choices. They can hit one button or they can hit another button. In this experiment in which they have multiple choices, now it's possible through this study using fMRI, functional MRI. In this case this study appeared in *The Journal of Nature and Neuroscience,* showed that there's some information that seems to predict the choice that's made up to 10 seconds in advance. So it's even more commitment before the awareness of a choice. So it's now 10 seconds of commitment beforehand. That sounds like a real demolishing of the concept of free will. But the caveat to this is that this neural activity is not super accurate at predicting what's going to happen, and so imagine if you have two choices, chance is 50 percent, it turns out this neural activity is only 60 or 70 percent accurate. So the current state of the research is that this preparatory activity, this predictive activity, that says that maybe we already kind of know what your choice is going to be, it seems to be reporting more of an inclination as opposed to hard evidence.

So what all this evidence together suggests is that as far as anyone can tell based on measuring neural activity, brain activity, either using EEG or fMRI, is that there's motor preparatory activity, and that motor preparatory activity perhaps causes the feeling of intention, that there are these processes that are rolling along that lead to a choice. Perhaps the moment when a decision is made can come before awareness of our own actions dawns upon us. If we step back from this and think about not picking over the fine tenths of a second, and the fine details of when we think we've made a decision, the net effect seems to be that our brains produce our actions, but part of the decision-making process in either the fMRI case or the EEG case, part of that decision-making process is complete before we're able to report it. So in that sense we're doers, not talkers.

For most of you this might be some kind of novel idea, the idea that there are aspects of leaning towards action, committing to an action, that are not really you picking your action, but more like your brain moving toward the action.

So that could be bothersome, it could be exciting, but I think it's a way of thinking about what free will really is.

Now let's step back a little bit. What does this kind of experiment mean for our conception of free will? I would propose that the problem of free will is mainly a difficult problem at a philosophical level and maybe that's the level at which it's worrisome, do I have free will or do I not? I think on a practical basis there's no real cause for worry. I think the practical implications of what we know about brain function are perhaps not as complicated. We can come up with practical definitions of free will that can guide our everyday lives, so here's one.

One practical definition of free will is based on predictability. Free will is a concept that's used to describe what an entire person does. If the behavior of an object, including a person, can be predicted with mathematical precision, it doesn't have free will. So if we consider an atom or a particle, those things don't have free will. According to one point of view, free will perhaps is ruled out by the idea that the output of our brains could somehow be predicted if we could know what was happening in every neuron, in every glial cell of our brain. But maybe a more useful interpretation is that when we think about something that's 100 billion neurons, and we're trying to predict what a complex system with that many components is doing, we can't do it. Nobody has done a complete computer simulation of even what a single neuron does biochemically and electrically, let alone the 100 billion neurons in an actual brain and the 10,000 connections each neuron makes.

There's a more fundamental issue, which I mentioned very briefly in an early lecture, which is that when synapses communicate, when a presynaptic action potential arrives and gets to the presynaptic terminal, it often does not lead to neurotransmitter release. Even single synapses are unpredictable. What that means is that single synapses fail. There's something thermodynamic about single synapses, that there is this fundamental uncertainty about whether neurotransmitter is released or not. So it's not just that our knowledge of what a brain is going to do is limited by knowledge by the state of all the cells and synapses. But in fact there are these unpredictable events that happen at the single synapse level. That doesn't mean that the whole system is unpredictable, but I'm just trying to give a sense of the difficulties involved in predicting what a system like the brain does. Predicting the details of what a whole brain will do then is basically impossible. So from a practical standpoint I would say that that's a functional definition of freedom, unpredictability, and perhaps of free will.

There's another question that sometimes comes up at this juncture which is this science fiction device of brain scanners that can read a person's mind. So I'm going to put a scanner on your head and detect what you're thinking. Is that even possible? Based on what I've said so far, I think you can guess where this is headed. At any moment many millions of neurons in your brain are generating electrical impulses. Reading what's happening in all of them at once is beyond the capability of any current technology. Even if you had such a recording, there's no way to convert those measurements to an interpretation of specific thoughts. This is a very hard problem.

There is a simpler example of this that's possible using current imaging technology. I've mentioned before that using fMRI it's possible for instance to see strong emotional responses in the form of increased activity in the amygdala. In general it's possible to get some information about what people are seeing by looking at brain activity patterns. For instance, if you have two competing images, let's say what I said before about one image being shown to the left eye and another one to the right, your conscious perception switches back and forth between those pictures. Researchers can identify patterns of activity that are associated with you being aware of either the left-eye stimulus or the right-eye stimulus. So it's possible, to an extent, to predict the consciously experienced stimulus. But it's only possible to do this after observing responses to hundreds of presentations of the images. And so one example of this that comes up in news articles, but also in science fiction, is the idea of a lie detector. Something that you put over your head and then goes off when you tell a lie.

Any attempt to design a brain scanner that could detect lies runs into similar problems. They have to be calibrated with hundreds of truth-telling events and lying events. That perhaps is a bit too much cooperation to expect for someone whose reward for helping the experimenter might be a prison sentence. I think the concept of a mind scanner, brain scanning lie detector, should probably not be taken seriously. I think there's no real concern about monitoring lies or truths, even with a million dollar instrument.

Now let's move on to another question of free will. Let's put away the tinfoil hat and let's step back a little bit. At some level the things I've talked about with knowing all the neurons, activity states in the brain, and brain scanning, perhaps these are technical points. It's not clear that these answer the hard question, the hard question being, even if we can't predict behavior practically, are we agents or are we robots? Who's in charge here? Recall that I told you lectures ago about Phineas Gage, and the fundamental lesson of the case of Phineas Gage is that brain injury can lead to changes in behavior. Remember that he was a hardworking guy who had prefrontal cortical damage and then that damage changed his life, changed his personality, changed something about his quintessential identity. It's a demonstration that our brains determine who we are. In general it's possible to understand moral behavior a little bit in this way, and I want to turn to a moral leader, the religious leader, the Dalai Lama. The Dalai Lama has posed the question of whether we should change the brain to influence behavior.

This is a guy who has been very interested in enlightenment, in ways that neuroscience can inform his practice of his religion. In 2005 he made a speech to the Annual Society for Neuroscience meeting and I got to ask him a question. There were thousands of people present and we got to ask down questions and they were passed forward, and my question was picked and the question is this. If neuroscience research could someday allow people to reach enlightenment by artificial means, such as drugs or surgery, would he be in favor of the treatment to alter people's moral behavior? And what he said was that if such a treatment had been available, it would have saved him time spent in meditation, freeing him up to do more good works. He even pointed at his own head saying that if he could remove bad thoughts by just removing a brain region, like Phineas Gage, he wanted to just cut it out. He made these stabbing motions at his own brain which was kind of disturbing, except that it came from somebody wearing the robes of a holy man, so that perhaps made it a little bit less frightening.

There's a caveat. He felt that such a treatment would only be acceptable if it left one's critical faculties intact. So for instance, this rules out the case of Phineas Gage, it also rules out the prefrontal lobotomy. This is a neurosurgical treatment invented by Egas Moniz, and popularized with great enthusiasm in the mid-20th century. This is a radical procedure that is in some ways not unlike what happened to Phineas Gage in which prefrontal lobes are disconnected from the rest of the brain. It was a very popular procedure in mental hospitals, primarily as a means of controlling violent and troublesome patients.

It did remove those impulses, but it also removed many functions that we associate with mental existence such as goal-directed action planning, motivation, complex reasoning, It has been abandoned as a surgical treatment.

The Dalai Lama's point about keeping one's critical faculties intact raises the point of moral responsibility for our actions. For instance, is it possible to separate our actions from our capacity for moral reasoning? There's a case study for this, and in some ways this case study is the opposite of what the Dalai Lama had in mind. There's a school teacher who was an intelligent and reasonable man who started acting strangely. He started collecting child pornography. He went to doctors, while at the doctor's office he couldn't stop leering at his nurse. He started making sexual advances towards his stepdaughter. He knew that these things were wrong so he had that level of moral awareness, but he couldn't stop himself. He told the doctor that he was afraid that he was going to commit a rape. And he had a terrible headache. A brain scan revealed that he had a tumor pushing on his orbital frontal cortex. This is a structure I've told you about before in regard to regulation of social behavior. When the tumor was removed, his sociopathic tendencies subsided and he went back to his normal self. His case points out that like emotional reactions and emotional decision making, moral understanding and awareness requires different brain areas from the ability to act morally.

So as neuroscience advances, then associations between brain structure and function will certainly expand. So one question is then, how do we start treating people who cannot act morally? How do we start dealing with moral offenses? For example, I'll pose you a few questions having to do with now our understanding of how brains generate behavior. So one question is, is life imprisonment the most effective means of punishing a 15-year-old whose prefrontal brain structures are not yet done developing? Recall that I talked about brain development happening through the 20s and not being complete until the 20s.

Is repair of a brain preferable to punishment? If we think about the Dalai Lama, perhaps at some point it'll be necessary to start thinking about his criterion of what would be ethical to do while leaving critical faculties intact? So these are questions of neuroscience and law, and neuroscience and moral behavior. Neuroscientists Jonathan Cohen and Josh Greene have said, "If neuroscience can change moral intuitions, then perhaps neuroscience can change the law."

One can start asking questions about other treatments, for instance Prozac, Ritalin, these are also treatments that change the brain. They're more subtle, but they are treatments that change the brain despite the fact that you don't go in with a surgical instrument. You're still doing something to change the brain. They seem innocuous, but they are things that we do that change our brains. I think it's a fairly important question to ask whether that's okay.

Now let me summarize what we've talked about today. First, we talked about consciousness. I've said that in any given moment we're consciously aware of only a small fraction of what we're doing or what's occurring around us, this attentional spotlight. I've also talked about philosophers and neuroscientists and their interests in qualia. I've talked about how the closest one can come experimentally is to look for a neural correlate of conscious experience. I've told you that even our own decisions are a target of conscious awareness, and what that means is that sometimes we become aware of simple decisions, or complex decision, only after our brains have made a commitment. We can sometimes stop actions, so free won't instead of free will.

From the standpoint of everyday life, conceptual difficulties with the question of free will are resolved in a practical sense with the concept that you're responsible for all your actions. You are your brain and your brain is responsible for your actions, as you are. Now, disease or injury can change you into a different person, so the understanding of that starts to raise questions in ethics and morality.

In the coming lectures what I'm going to start talking about is other deep aspects of identity and experience. I'm going to talk about extreme experiences such as near-death experiences, and also spirituality.

Near-Death and Other Extreme Experiences
Lecture 34

Out-of-body experiences happen in about 10% of the healthy population ... once or twice in a lifetime.

Mountaineers have long known to watch for the dangers of their sport, in particular when they're at high altitude, and they know to watch out for things that can happen in thin air. Many of the effects that they observe are attributable to the reduced supply of oxygen to the brain. At 2,500 meters or higher, some mountaineers report perceiving unseen companions, light emanating from themselves or from their body parts or the body parts of others, a second body like their own, or a figure where there is none. They suddenly feel such emotions as fear. The physical effects of mountain climbing, such as low oxygen, intense exertion, and stress, may account for these phenomena—they seem to increase, for instance, the likelihood of a seizure. Out-of-body experiences happen in about 10% of the healthy population, who have them once or twice in a lifetime. Evidence supports the idea that out-of-body experiences depend on the temporal parietal junction.

The temporal parietal junction of the brain seems to be involved in spatial self-perception and, thus, may be a candidate for understanding these phenomena. The parietal and temporal lobes sit on the brain surface close to the somata (body) sensory cortex, near where auditory and visual information comes in; thus, it seems well positioned to integrate

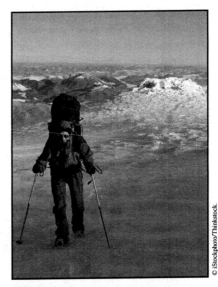

© iStockphoto/Thinkstock.

Mountain climbers can experience mental anomalies due to reduced supply of oxygen to the brain.

information from these sensory areas. There is also good evidence that this brain region is important for representations of the body.

Visions and visitations seem to be associated with the temporal lobe. The temporal and **parietal lobes** of the cortex are involved in visual and face processing, as well as emotional events. Oxygen deprivation is likely to interfere with activity in neural structures, and the temporal and parietal lobes seem particularly susceptible to oxygen deprivation. This association between oxygen deprivation and paranormal experiences may be associated with either temporal parietal seizures or temporal lobe seizures.

The phenomenon of haunted houses, common in the 19th and early 20th centuries, is associated with using gas for house lighting: a source of carbon monoxide emission. Carbon monoxide binds to hemoglobin, the molecule that carries oxygen in the blood and leads to oxygen deprivation to the brain. Reports of haunted houses have diminished considerably now that gas is no longer used to light houses.

Near-death experiences are characterized by the feeling of leaving your physical body and seeing your life flashing before you. They have been estimated to happen in 9–18% of persons near the point of death. One possible explanation is that general oxygen deprivation can lead to widespread activity throughout the brain, and it's easy to imagine that this kind of activity could account for accelerated thought processes.

All the different kinds of brain activity triggered by various events, from seizures to dreams, require the brain to convert them into a storyline. One unifying explanation is that the brain is engaging in some kind of confabulation to piece together a story from incomplete or highly unusual data. ∎

Important Term

parietal lobe: A cortical lobe bordered by the central sulcus of Rolando anteriorly, the parieto-occipital sulcus posteriorly, and the Sylvian (lateral) fissure inferiorly.

1. What common factor(s) may underlie visions at altitude and haunted-house visitations?

2. How might low blood oxygen during a near-death experience lead to the feeling of "life review"?

Near-Death and Other Extreme Experiences
Lecture 34—Transcript

Welcome back. In the last lecture we talked about consciousness and free will, and that's a subject that perhaps you would've expected to be right at the edge of neuroscience. So now what we're going to do is we're going to talk about a subject that might seem to be outside the range of science altogether, namely paranormal phenomena. So in this lecture what we're going to do is we're going to talk about near death and other extreme experiences. We're going to talk about extreme experiences, and we're going to talk about things such as out-of-body experiences, meditation, religious visions, and we're going to connect them to everyday unusual experiences, namely dreams. Let's start with some of these extreme experiences that you or I are unlikely to experience in everyday life.

One category of strange paranormal phenomena is reported by mountain climbers at altitude. Different kinds of athletes report strange things happening to them when they're in the zone and they're doing extreme things. But one exceptional group is mountain climbers. Mountaineers have long known to watch for the dangers of their sport, in particular when they're at high altitude, and they know to watch out for things that can happen in thin air. An example is acute mountain sickness which can occur above altitudes of 2,500 meters, about 8,000 feet. Many of the effects that they observe are attributable to the reduced supply of oxygen to the brain. So, for example, reaction times are measurably reduced at altitudes as low as 1,500 meters, about 5,000 feet. But at 2,500 meters or higher, some mountaineers report perceiving unseen companions. They report seeing light emanating from themselves, from their body parts, or perhaps the body parts of others. Sometimes they see a second body like their own or they see a figure where there's nobody. They suddenly feel emotions like fear. These are all things that happen to mountain climbers.

Now, what could possibly cause these strange events? It turns out that there are physical events during mountain climbing that, for neurological reasons, could be predictive of these strange events. They are, namely as I've mentioned, low oxygen, but also intense exertion and stress. These are physical events that seem to increase, for instance, the likelihood of a seizure.

It appears to be the case that there are parts of the brain that are involved in self-perception and in our maps in our perceptions of the world, that could contribute to what these mountain climbers are experiencing. So let's think about this. It turns out that one brain region that seems like it might be a candidate for what's going on in these mountain climbers is a part of the brain called the "temporal parietal junction."

The temporal parietal junction is a site that seems to be involved in spacial self-perception. Let's look at where it is in on the brain. If we look at the parietal lobe and the temporal lobe on the brain surface, they sit in the brain in a place that's seen to be a good place for multisensory integration of the body for self-processing, for integration of body-related information. If you look at where the temporal parietal junction is, it's at a place that's not too far from the somata sensory cortex, which is up at the parietal lobe near where the frontal lobe is, it's near where auditory information comes in, and it's also near where visual information comes in. So this temporal parietal region seems to be well positioned to integrate different kinds of information from these different sensory areas, somata sensory, auditory, and visual.

So it's well located for that, and it turns out that there is good evidence that this brain region is important for representations of the body. There are other brain regions as well, so for instance if you look closer to the visual cortex, there are regions such as the extrastriate body area. This is a brain area that seems to be respond selectively to the sight of human bodies and of body parts. It's also in an area where you can find neural activity that corresponds to your own movement and also the movement of others. This is some kind of mirror function, so recall that we've talked about mirror neurons. This is a place where one can find mirror functionality.

It turns out to be possible to induce out-of-body experiences in these brain regions. So, for example, in epileptic patients—we're back to epileptic patients who have electrodes put into them in order to find out where their seizures begin—it's possible to then put in these electrode arrays to record and it's also possible to stimulate. It's possible to stimulate in various regions in the temporal and parietal lobes and to induce an illusory shadow person. So it's possible to find a place on the brain, in the left hemisphere as it turns out, that prompts the creepy feeling that somebody is close by.

So it's possible to induce this feeling that perhaps your body is here and there's another body behind you. Or perhaps if you're sitting upright, there's another body behind you, and it's even possible for there to be details, for instance, that the perception is that the body is behind you and holding you back and preventing you from moving. So it's possible to stimulate in the temporal parietal junction and find regions that seem to trigger out-of-body experiences.

Now let's back up and ask a question. When do out-of-body experiences happen? Out-of-body experiences, as I've mentioned, are an experience in which you see your own body, and you either perceive a body outside your own, or you experience the world from a location outside your own body. It turns out that out-of-body experiences happen in about 10 percent of the healthy population. They're reported in most cultures. This 10 percent of the population perhaps will experience an out-of-body experience once or twice in a lifetime. So if you think about that, that is a large number of people, it means that you have a 1 in 10 chance, even if you're not epileptic or suffer other neurological damage, of experiencing one of these out-of-body experiences. It turns out that these experiences also happen in epileptics and in cases of brain damage.

Evidence supports the idea that this kind of out-of-body experience seems to depend on the temporal parietal junction. I've already talked about electrophysiology in epileptics. It's also possible to look in people with lesions in the brain and it's also possible to trigger an out-of-body experience with transcranial magnetic stimulation. So it's possible to alter brain activity with a magnetic field that's placed outside the head to induce electrical activity in the brain and cause an out-of-body experience. It has even been visualized using fMRI. So it's been possible to take a person and put that person in a scanner, and do fMRI recording, and see neural correlates of out-of-body experience. So it's possible to see brain activity that corresponds to the experience of having your body go outside your body.

We can also ask the question can we induce this in a normal person? I've told you that 1 out of 10 people experience an out-of-body experience during their lifetime, is it possible to experimentally induce this? It turns out that it is possible. It's possible to do it both in a limb and also with the whole body.

So for instance, a very interesting experiment has been done by colleagues of mine, Matt Botvinick and John Cohen. They've done an experiment in which they can cause people to feel that a hand that's made of rubber is their own hand, and this is the way they did the experiment. They seated subjects with their left arm resting on a small table and a standing screen was positioned beside the arm to hide it from the subject's view, and then instead, a life-sized rubber model of a left hand and arm was placed on the table directly in front of the subject. The subject sat with his or her eyes fixed on the artificial hand, and then what the experimenters did is they used two small paintbrushes, one to stroke the rubber hand and one to stroke the subject's hidden hand. These were synchronized as closely as possible. So this is a very simple experiment where you brush the rubber hand and you brush the real hand in sync with one another.

After 10 minutes of this, subjects were asked to complete a questionnaire on what they experienced. What they experienced was the subjective sense that the hand on the table was their own hand. They experienced the sight of touch, as if their own hand had been touched. So they started getting the sense that this rubber hand, which was at a distance from their own hand, was part of their hand. They even had the subjective experience that their hand was farther away from their body. So this gets to the feeling of an out-of-body experience where their subjective feeling of where there hand was, was moved by this simple manipulation of stroking their real hand and a rubber hand that they were looking at. So the visual information of looking at an artificial hand could be used to guide the representation of the body.

It turns out that in more recent years this has also been done with the body surface. In this more recent experiment that was just done a few years ago, it was possible to do the same thing or a very similar thing with a body surface. In this case it was an experiment in which it was possible to induce the sensation of looking at your own body from behind. So in this case it's an experiment where you look at a virtual body and the virtual body is touched in sync with your own body being touched like that. So again, integration of two pieces of information, the feeling of touch and the sight of a virtual body being touched. This joint stimulation of visual plus tactile sense was able to generate a sense that your own body was outside your body. So it's possible, with very simple techniques, to generate an out-of-body experience. In fact, you could probably try this at home if you chose to. This is an example of what seems to be a fairly exotic experience that can be induced by things ranging from epileptic seizure to something like simple touch.

Now let's turn to another kind of phenomenon, the phenomena of visions and visitations. Visions and visitations are things that happen, again, under sometimes extreme conditions and sometimes under non-extreme conditions. In this case these experiences seem to be associated now with temporal lobe epilepsy. So now we've moved from the temporal parietal junction now to the temporal lobe. When we look at temporal lobe seizures, there are certain kinds of things that happen. So these seizures typically generate subjective experience that's related to things that are found in the temporal lobe. So now I've talked about the temporal and parietal lobes of the cortex being involved in visual and face processing, and also emotional events, and I've also talked about risk factors for seizures. I've mentioned oxygen deprivation. It turns out that oxygen deprivation is likely to interfere with activity in neural structures. It seems to be that the temporal and parietal lobes are particularly susceptible to oxygen deprivation. There's something about those regions, large neurons, there's something there that that makes them more susceptible to deprivation of oxygen.

It also turns out that in the case of the temporal lobe, which I'm going to give you examples of, temporal lobe seizures are triggered more easily under conditions that elevate endorphins, for instance, conditions of high stress. So we're back to the mountain climbers. In addition to mountain climbers, there are other groups that also experience strange experiences at altitude. So this association between oxygen deprivation and paranormal experiences has occurred in other groups, and another group that these events have happen to is people who experience intense religious experiences. So it turns out that temporal lobe seizures are often associated with intense religious experiences, and here are some examples. These experiences include feeling the presence of God, feeling an unseen presence, a feeling that one is in heaven, and seeing emanations of light. Remember I talked about mountain climbers and how mountain climbers often saw emanations of light from other people. Here again we have emanations of light, this time perhaps associated with either temporal parietal seizures or temporal lobe seizures.

It's possible to find examples of this kind of phenomenon in stories from the three major monotheistic religions practiced today: Judaism, Christianity, and Islam. All three of these religions involve special visions that occurred at great heights, and let's think about some examples. If up look in the Old Testament, Moses encountered a voice emanating from a burning bush on top of Mount Sinai. A voice coming from a burning bush. Jesus' followers witnessed the transfiguration on what was probably Mt. Hermon, and this is an event in which light was seen emanating from Jesus. Third example—in Islam, Muhammad, in his conversion, was on top of a mountain called Mt. Hira, also called Jibal An-Noor. He was visited by an angel who pressed on his chest and instructed him to recite. He said I can't, and the angel said you must recite. And he felt fear and he felt this crushing feeling on his chest.

It turns out that many of these spiritual experiences have common features. They include feeling and hearing a presence; seeing a figure; seeing lights, sometimes emanating from a person; and the sensation of fear. These, in fact, overlap quite a lot with the events that I told you about before in the case of mountain climbers, events that are associated with temporal lobe epilepsy. These visions are just three examples of a broad category of mystical experience. If you look through religious experiences that people have had around the world, it is quite common to see visitations and visions that happen under extreme conditions. For example, in Mexico there is the peasant Juan Diego who ran across Tepeyac Hill in Guadalupe. When he was running across that hill, the Virgin Mary appeared to him and said, you should build a church here. In this vision he saw roses, he saw the Blessed Virgin, and this is the beginning of the Virgin of Guadalupe. It turns out in addition to being on mountaintops, religious visions often also occur under stressful conditions. So there is a commonly observed phenomenon in which stressful conditions also are conditions under which religious visions can occur. As a general rule, visions are then associated not only with mountains, but also other remote areas. So if we think about deserts, for instance, deserts are a place where it is often reported that people have religious visions.

Seizures are thought to have caused religious visions in many historical figures, examples include St. Teresa of Ávila and also St. Therese of Lisieux. And the case of St. Therese of Lisieux is a very interesting example. This is a woman who took Holy Orders, joined a convent at a very early age, but also was reported at a very early age to have tremors. So she had tremors, these tremors turned into clenched teeth, and the inability to talk. Of course these are signs that we now know as being signs of seizure. She was born in 1873, and so very early in her life, in 1882, a doctor named Gayral diagnosed that she reacted "to an emotional frustration with a neurotic attack." So this is something that she observed at a very early age. Also just the next year she gazed at a statue of the blessed Virgin Mary and she reported that the Virgin turned and smiled at her. And she in fact was canonized as a result of this apparent miracle.

Temporal lobe seizures may have triggered conversions of previously nonreligious people and these are also found in the record. One example is the Apostle Paul on his way to Damascus. Another example is the American Joseph Smith who's the Founder of the Church of Latter Day Saints. So these are examples of possible cases of temporal lobe epilepsy associated with religious visions.

Now I want to turn to a very different kind of paranormal experience, one that is more modern. It's the phenomenon of haunted houses. Haunted houses are phenomena that were observed in the early 20th century and perhaps are less frequently observed today, much less frequently observed today. The phenomena of haunted houses is associated with events that I think at this point you will recognize as being fairly familiar, and let me describe some of the things that are reported as going with haunted houses. The sound of footsteps, a crushing feeling in the chest, an invisible presence, and fear. In addition to all these phenomena, another thing that's observe in haunted houses is sometimes the sudden and inexplicable death of the occupants of the house.

There are some good records of haunted houses in the historical literature and it turns out that there's a classic paper from 1921 written by an ophthalmologist named Wilmer who's the founder of a famous eye institute, the Wilmer Eye Institute at Johns Hopkins University. He wrote in 1921 of accounts of cases that are strange, that resemble haunted house visitations, and he quotes in full a story, a chronicle, by a Mrs. B, about what happened in her house. I'll just tell you exactly what she wrote. She wrote, for instance, "One morning I heard footsteps in the room over my head. I hurried up the stairs. To my surprise, the room was empty. I passed into all the rooms on that floor and then to the floor above. I found that I was the only person in that part of the house." So that was something that she observed. She also said, "Many mornings when going downstairs or through the halls, I would notice an order of gas." And we'll come to that.

She and her family also reported severe headaches, feeling weak and tired, her children grew pale and listless. Her houseplants died. Her husband reported being woken many nights by the sound of a bell ringing. One evening he woke up and found that he thought the fire department was going to put out a fire down the street. He heard a terrific clanging, and he went outside and he found a quiet deserted street. One day Mrs. B found that she was walking down the hallway and saw a figure, saw a woman down the hallway, and wondered who that woman was. She looked and then looked again and it turned out to be just a mirror and herself. At another time, Mrs. B's house servant reported complaining thinking that her husband was sitting on top of her at night crushing the breath out of her. So all these were strange things, and in fact, the house servant was convinced that the house was haunted, and so these are all classic signs of haunted house visitation. So they called a researcher and the researcher's assistant came over and looked around the house and investigated and "found the furnace in a very bad condition, the combustion being imperfect. The fumes, instead of going up the chimney, were pouring gases of carbon monoxide into the rooms."

Let's go back. The odor of gas. It turns out that one common phenomenon associated with using gas for house lighting is the emission of carbon monoxide, and it turns out that carbon monoxide binds to hemoglobin, this is the molecule that carries the oxygen in the blood. Carbon monoxide binds to hemoglobin very tightly, more tightly in fact than oxygen does, and so in fact, carbon monoxide leads to oxygen deprivation to the brain. Perhaps this sounds familiar, right, oxygen deprivation to the brain leading to, for instance, temporal lobe epilepsy, maybe temporal parietal lobe epilepsy. Now it turns out that reports of haunted houses have in fact diminished considerably now that gas is no longer used to light houses.

Now let's turn to a very strange experience, an experience known as "near-death experiences." Near-death experiences include this feeling that's called "dissociation." Dissociation is defined as separation of thoughts, feelings, or experiences, from the normal stream of consciousness and memory and daily experience, this feeling of being separated from your own consciousness. In particular, dissociation is quite often seen in near-death experience. A near-death experience includes, for instance, the feeling of leaving your physical body, transcending the boundaries of the self, and the ordinary confines of time and space. Near-death experiences have been reported in many cultures and are associated with some very characteristic phenomena that include accelerated thought processes, and what's called "life review." So this feeling that your life is flashing before you, and a feeling of peace and joy and a feeling of being out of the body. Near-death experiences have been estimated to happen in 9 to18 percent of persons near the point of death, and there have been studies of near-death experiences.

So what could cause near-death experiences? It turns out that very recently there has been a study looking at brain activity at the time of death. It has been possible to record EEG activity, also muscle activity, and in this case the EEG activity is the one thing that can be measured because they're emotionless sedated patients who are near death. It's been possible to look at brain activity at the time of death. What's seen in these patients is a surge of activity, and the surge of activity takes the form of an EEG signal, the signal that reflects the synchronized activity of many neurons together in the brain. The surge of activity lasts for several minutes. Now, what could be causing this?

Remember at the beginning of this course I talked about how the brain needs a lot of energy, how oxygen and glucose are needed to maintain voltage differences across the membrane. In particular, oxygen and glucose, this 15 watts of power, are needed to power the sodium-potassium pump, this pump that moves sodium out of the cell and potassium into the cell. It turns out at the point of death and near death it is quite commonly observed that the blood pressure of these patients goes to zero, and in fact, so does their blood oxygen. It's known that cases of low blood oxygen are associated with a rise in potassium levels. So what happens is that potassium levels which are previously pumped, those potassium levels can change, and the change in potassium levels would have a probable consequence of changing the voltage across neuronal membranes. What that means is that the normal neuronal membranes change in how excitable they are. What's likely to happen in such a case is that there's activity that's triggered, perhaps a burst of activity, before it's no longer possible for the neurons to fire. One possibility then is that general oxygen deprivation can lead to widespread activity throughout the brain. It's easy to imagine that this kind of activity, this wave of excitation, this deprivation of oxygen and change in potassium levels, could in fact account for accelerated thought processes and could in fact account for your life flashing before your eyes. Imagine generalized brain activity all throughout the brain happening in short order, imagine you trying to make sense of that activity. It's easy to imagine that this could account for the subjective sense that you're recalling many things and your life is flashing before your eyes.

Now let's think about another strange experience. Let's go back now to something I talked about earlier which is the experience of drug experiences. People often take drugs in order to experience altered states of reality. One very famous drug in this case is a drug known as acid, also known as LSD. It turns out that LSD is a serotonin receptor blocker, specifically it blocks type 2 serotonin receptors, and it turns out that LSD has a variety of effects. It alters sensory perception, it alters vision, it distorts your field of view, it gives you a lot of strange sensory experiences. Of course these strange sensory experiences need to be interpreted. Now that we've talked a lot about how the brain is constantly in the business of interpreting what happens in the world, it's easy to imagine that these alterations in sensory experience then have to be interpreted by the brain in terms of what really happened. If you read accounts of what LSD does, LSD brings out amazingly vivid imagery and appears to allow thoughts and perceptions that would otherwise be inaccessible. For instance, the poet Anne Waldman once described to me a trip in which she stood in front of a full-length mirror and she said she saw herself aging from a little girl to an old woman continuously. She saw herself at every stage of her life separately and together all at once. This is very clearly a very strange experience, one in which there is something that happened in her brain in which she experienced a very strange sensory or perceptual event. This recollection then got turned into some perception in which she looked at herself in the mirror and saw all these things happening.

Here's another example, and this comes back to everyday life, the example is dreams. Dreams have been suggested by neuroscientists to be the reactivation of brain activity as we sleep. So as we sleep our brains are not receiving input from the outside world, but are still active. It has been suggested that what dreams are is basically reactivation of brain activity, perhaps random reactivation of brain activity patterns, basically letting the brain run loose and engaging these acts of spontaneous activity.

Now let's think about what we've talked about in previous lectures about what the brain is doing. The brain is an interpreter. It's still trying to interpret what's going on. In the case of LSD there's sensory alteration; in the case of a dream the input is very different. In all these cases, everything I've talked about here, out-of-body experiences, temporal lobe epilepsy, visions, mountain climbers, now LSD and dreams—all these are different kinds of brain activity that are triggered by various events. The brain needs to convert these kinds of events into a story line in interpretation of what's going on in the world. So one unifying explanation for all these kinds of events is that the brain is engaging in perhaps some kind of lying or confabulation where it's trying to take information and figure out what's happening. It's trying to piece together a story from incomplete data or data that is highly unusual and convert that into a coherent storyline and figure out what's going on.

Let's summarize what we've talked about. We've talked about out-of-body and altered body perceptual experiences. I've told you about how these experiences can arise from disruption in temporal and parietal brain regions. These events can be triggered by a variety of events: lack of oxygen, intense exertion, physical or emotional stress, the stress of some extreme thing happening to you. Unusual perceptual experiences of course can be quite memorable, and in fact in some cases they can even trigger religious conversions. These very strange experiences then, while paranormal, can perhaps in some sense be explained or accounted for by these events that are physical phenomena happening within our brains. So I think these paranormal phenomena perhaps are getting drawn a little bit more into the realm of phenomena that perhaps we can study, one that is less mysterious, but perhaps no less remarkable.

In the next lecture what I'd like to do is turn away from these phenomena and start considering the phenomena of spirituality and also religious experience.

Spirituality and Religion
Lecture 35

The ability to cooperate and to compete with our fellow beings may have set the stage for forming religious mental constructs.

When Buddhists talk about meditation, they divide it into two major categories: stilling the mind, or stabilizing meditation, and a process of understanding, meditating on an object or meditating on an idea—discursive meditation. Investigators have studied the first category in Buddhist monks who are well practiced in the process of objectless meditation by measuring patterns of electrode activity. At first, those patterns were no different from those of volunteers who were meditating for the first time. But when asked to generate a feeling of compassion, the brains of experienced practitioners began varying in a coherent rhythmic oscillation, suggesting that many neural structures were firing in synchrony with one another, a phenomenon called gamma rhythm. Several types of rhythm seem to get stronger with experience in novices who learn meditation, which suggests that the capacity is at least partly trainable. Similarly, prayer might benefit the person doing the praying just as meditation benefits or changes the brain patterns of these Buddhist monks. That is to say, prayer might benefit us in a process that transforms our mental state.

Anthropologists have studied religion around the world

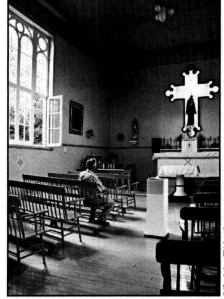

Prayer, like meditation, can change the practitioner's brain state.

and found that having religion offers advantages—in particular, religion is a powerful early instrument of group social bonding, and it has been suggested that this social bonding presents some kind of competitive advantage to help the group survive. Religion is a highly sophisticated cultural phenomenon involving many components. Brain capabilities important for forming and transmitting religious beliefs include the search for causes and effects, social reasoning, and language and the cultural transmission of information.

Social communication requires such structures as the amygdala, which is intimately involved in deriving the emotional significance of objects and faces and, thus, is critical in giving the brain access to the mental states of others. These forms of social complexity seem to be related to the size of the **cerebral cortex**. The ability to cooperate and to compete with our fellow beings may have set the stage for forming religious mental constructs.

The notion that accumulated ideas could be modified, allowing a doctrine and a dogma to be communicated and preserved from generation to generation, requires language, an aspect that is less well understood from a neuroscientific standpoint but important in terms of what makes religious belief possible. Our capacity for language allows our search for causes and effects to take on a new dimension in the form of narrative.

Any eventual neuroscientific explanation of how we form narratives is likely to address how narratives lead us to believe a story. For example, how exactly would an omniscient omnipotent being run the world? One point of view is that God would put every detail in place. But another point of view might be that God works through amazing processes, such as natural selection and brains. Rather than having to supervise everything from moment to moment, perhaps God launched natural processes to ensure the functioning of creation. In this respect, neuroscience is a way of understanding more deeply the world around us. ■

Important Term

cerebral cortex: The outer sheet or mantle of cells covering the hemispheres.

1. What brain capacities are necessary in order to be able to form a belief in God?

2. In light of known brain mechanisms, how might prayer have an effect, and in whose brain?

Spirituality and Religion
Lecture 35—Transcript

Welcome back. In the last lecture we talked about extreme experiences, near-death experiences, temporal parietal lobe seizures. Some of those experiences were connected with religious experience, and so it seems appropriate now to tackle a fairly large topic, the topic of spirituality and religion. So what I'd like to do in this lecture is talk about spiritual experience, talk about the things that happen in our brains as we have spiritual religious experiences. And also spend a little bit of time thinking about what brain capacities make it possible for us to be religious in the first place. So those are the main goals for what I'm going to be doing in the coming lecture.

Let's first talk about the neuroscience of having an intense religious experience. Let's take, as an example, a phenomenon that has been studied in some detail over the last few years, and namely that phenomena is meditation. One person who has taken a lot of interest in the neuroscience of religious experience is the Dalai Lama. The Dalai Lama has taken the view that Buddhist doctrine is not unchanging, but in fact that when scientific discoveries come into conflict with Buddhist doctrine, the doctrine must give way. He has also had a strong interest in exploring the neuromechanisms underlying meditation. It turns out that the Dalai Lama is a very technically minded person and has always been very interested in tinkering with engines, with motors, and he has a natural interest in science. When Buddhists talk about meditation, including the Dalai Lama, meditation is divided into two major categories of what constitutes meditation. So, despite the fact that we use one word for these things, one major category is meditation that is focused with the goal of stilling the mind, so stabilizing meditation. Another type of meditation is an active cognitive process, and this is a process of understanding. So, for instance discursive meditation, meditating on an object or meditating on an idea.

The first pass that neuroscientists have taken at studying meditation has focused on the first category. This consist of studies looking at brain activity in highly skilled practitioners of stabilizing Buddhist meditation. These are people who spend their lives stabilizing their minds, practicing meditation for many hours a day. These people were evaluated by a group of scientists, and one of the scientists was someone with a Ph.D. in molecular biology who has since joined the Chechen monastery in Nepal as a disciple. What has been done with these people is that Buddhist monks have been engaged in meditation and then their brain electrical patterns have been measured, and here's how the experiment was done.

The investigators took eight long-term practitioners of Tibetan Buddhist meditation away from their normal practice, which as I said, is spending all day in meditative retreats. So these are people who are very well practiced in the process of objectless meditation. What was done was electrodes were placed on their heads to measure patterns of electrode activity. First those patterns were no different than those of volunteers who are meditating for the very first time. So naïve volunteers and experienced meditators seemed to have similar brain activity patterns.

The difference came when the monks were asked to generate a feeling of compassion. As I said before, this is an undirected feeling. They were asked to, on command, generate a feeling of compassion not directed at any particular being, but just in general. This is a state that is known as "objectless meditation." What was seen was very interesting. What was seen in the brains of these experienced practitioners was that under these conditions the activity of their brains began varying in a coherent rhythmic matter. This coherent rhythmic oscillation suggested that many neural structures were firing in synchrony with one another. Recall earlier in this course I told you that EEG is the summed activity of many neurons at once. So when neurons fire together or generate synaptic activity at the same time, when that occurs in synchrony then that synchrony generates a signal that you can pick up when you put electrodes on the scalp.

In these practitioners what was observed was that there was a synchronized signal that was increased at rates of 25 to 40 Hz, 24 to 40 oscillations per second, and this is a rhythm known as "gamma band oscillations," and it's associated with synaptic activity. What was seen in some cases was that the gamma rhythms in these monk's brain signals were the largest ever seen in normal people. The only time that such signals had ever been seen was in pathological states such as seizures. Yet these were not epileptics, these were practiced monks. In contrast, the naïve meditators, recall that there was a control group, couldn't generate much additional gamma rhythm at all.

How brains generate synchronization is not well understood. But gamma rhythms have been observed to be greater under certain kinds of mental activity, so for instance, mental activity such as attending closely to a sensory stimulus, so during attention, also during maintenance of working memory. So there are conditions under which gamma band rhythm is enhanced, and this increased gamma band rhythm might be a key component of the heightened awareness reported by monks.

This is interesting, these monks have a large amount of gamma band that they can generate, and the question arises, are they born with a natural ability to generate a lot of brain synchrony or is it something that comes with practice? Several types of rhythm seem to get stronger with experience in novices who learn meditation. What that suggests is that the capacity is at least partly trainable. Recall that these are people who spend all day doing it, and so it would not be terribly surprising that what they're really doing is in fact training their brains to get into a state that includes something that can be measurable by a physical experimental method, namely EEG.

Another kind of meditation, discursive meditation, has also been investigated. It has been possible to identify regions of the brain that are active during discursive meditation, and now we're talking fMRI, functional MRI, to get good spatial resolution of which parts of the brain are active. In particular the kind of meditation that has been studied is the second kind of meditation that I mentioned, and this involves focused attention on a visualized image. These people are asked to focus on an image and think about that image and contemplate it. Under this condition the anterior cingulate and the prefrontal areas of the cortex were very active, and these are areas of the brain that we've heard about a lot in conjunction with executive function and also with directing one's attention.

It turns out that these brain regions are very active when Carmelite nuns are asked to recall the feeling of mystical union with God. So Carmelite nuns constitute a holy order in which they experience union with God as if they are married to God. This work fits with the involvement of these regions in attention. These are people who are asked to engage in focused attention and specifically focus on an image that they have in their minds. This is very interesting not only from the standpoint of Buddhism, but of course Catholicism in the case of the Carmelite nuns. It probably would have been of interest to Pope John Paul II. Recall that Pope John Paul II said, in reference to science and Catholic doctrine, he said that they were both true, they were both compatible with one another, and he said, "Truth cannot contradict truth." So there's a general feeling among these religious leaders that there should not be a conflict between scientific knowledge and what happens in the investigation of religion.

Now what I'd like to do is turn to another kind of event, something that happens in people's everyday lives, namely I want to talk just briefly about prayer. These findings on meditation perhaps imply an interesting twist on the neuroscience of prayer. When one reads about prayer in the scientific literature, or in say, literature regarding alternative medicine, so far what has been studied in the literature is the effects of prayer on the object of the prayer. For instance, if people are asked to pray for someone who is sick at a long distance, that's a phenomenon known as distance healing. When these kinds of things have been studied, those studies have been negative. There has not been a demonstrative effect of prayer on patients who are at a distance. Now let's turn that around a little bit. Let's talk about the neuroscience of praying in the mind, in the brain of the person who's doing the praying.

One might imagine, based on what I've told you about meditation, that prayer might benefit the person doing the praying just as meditation benefits or changes the brain patterns of these Carmelite nuns and of these Buddhist monks. That is to say, it might be that prayer benefits you in a process that transforms your mental state, as opposed to this other phenomenon of distance healing. So that's an interesting take on it. Recall that when I talked about left-handedness and left-handed athletes, there's some question about whether left-handed athletes have an advantage. People have always been very interested in the advantages enjoyed by the left-handed athletes, but there's evidence that in fact the advantage is in the brains of their opponents. This is now the converse experience, prayer benefiting the person who's doing the praying.

I want to make a general point about the neuroscience of strange experiences, of unusual experiences. Here's a major lesson about the neuroscience of spiritual experiences. I know that it's often the case that people talk about science as being opposed in some way to spiritual experiences, opposed to religious belief. But I think it's important to think about these things in the following context. Learning about what's going on in the brain during a spiritual experience does not necessarily impact one's religious belief at all. I would say that like the Pope, and like the Dalai Lama, I would take the position that knowing more about how prayer affects the brain doesn't necessarily keep you from praying. In fact, it's entirely possible that understanding these things might make you pray more. Knowing that a certain kind of temporal lobe activity is correlated with intense religious experience, as we talked about on the last lecture, does not explain away the religious experience unless you want it to. So your agency in choosing religion, choosing what to believe, is not directly affected by knowing more about brain mechanisms. It's a form of investigating nature, of understanding nature a little bit more, understanding yourself a little bit more.

Conversely, if you are not a person of faith, many religious phenomena perhaps make more sense in light of these findings. So if you are not a believer, many of these phenomena will often make a lot of sense. In that respect, I would propose that neuroscience is an adjunct to one's personal beliefs not unlike its relationship to other areas concerning human values. For instance, as we saw on a previous lecture, on philosophy, consciousness, and free will.

Now that I've talked about these questions of spiritual experience, about meditation, and prayer, maybe this is good preparatory information to lead us into a rather large question; and the large question is that of religion itself. There have been attempted explanations of religion, of what it is that religion is, from the standpoint of different kinds of investigation. So one major point of view that has been in the news the last few years is the view taken by some biologists, and the biologists take the view that religious beliefs are non-rational beliefs, beliefs that do not correspond with empirical reality. There are people who have taken this position, for instance there's the evolutionary biologist Richard Dawkins who has written a book called *The God Delusion*. He's sort of a bomb thrower who has taken the point of view that religion is a purely biological construct. Another example is the philosopher Daniel Dennett who has written a book called *Breaking the Spell: Religion as a Natural Phenomenon.* So that's one point of view about what religion is, and some people have taken that point of view.

Here's another scientific view about what religion is. Anthropologists have studied religion around the world and they found that there are advantages that come from having religion. In particular, anthropologists have noted that religion is a powerful early instrument of group social bonding. So if we think about what is advantageous to a group, a kin group, or a tribe, it might be advantageous to have shared values, to have shared beliefs about your own group and about others. It has been suggested by anthropologists that in fact this social bonding, whatever form it takes, presents some kind of competitive advantage to help that group survive better. So, religion is one of a number of beliefs and of a set of values that can lead to increased social cohesion.

These are prior stabs that people have taken at understanding what religion is from the standpoint of particular scientific disciplines. Now what I'd like to do is back up a little bit and talk about elements of religion and think about what brain capacities seem to be necessary for forming a religious belief. Without taking a position on exactly what it means for brains to have those capacities, but just to point out what the capacities are that are necessary for religious belief. Let's think about common elements of religion.

Religion is a highly sophisticated cultural phenomenon, one of the most sophisticated phenomenon known culturally, and it involves many components. So here are the components. Religions typically involve elaborate cognitive representation of a supernatural force that cannot be seen. This force reduces harm, brings about justice, or provides us with moral structure. This force also sets standards. These standards are thought by the adherents of whatever religion it is to establish the same standards of morals, social norms, and religious rituals that in some cases apply to all of us. These are common features of religion.

Now let's think about what brain capabilities are important for the formation of these religious beliefs, and also for the transmission of religious beliefs.

Here are some of the components. First, one component is the search for causes and effects. I've talked about this in the context of theory of mind, the idea that many animals will go around in the world looking for causes and effects, something that happens and then clouds form and then rain falls. That would be an example of cause and effect.

Another capacity that seems to be necessary for religious belief is social reasoning. Recall that social reasoning is a capacity that is unusually highly developed in humans. Remember that one of the core skills of the human brain is the ability to reason about people and motives, this thing that I've talked about called "theory of mind" when I talked about the social brain.

Lastly, a third capacity that's necessary for forming and transmitting religious belief is language and the cultural transmission of information.

Consequences of these capacities. These key features of mental function that are part of religious belief as they pertain to religious belief are, then, our ability to make causal inferences and abstractions, to infer unseen intentions. When we infer unseen intentions they are entities that are unseen, they could be a person, they could be someone out of sight. But they could also be the intentions of a deity who has views about what we ought to be doing. So if we think about how these play into religion we can think about how they relate to religious explanations. One component is imputing intentionality to events. When we look for intentionality of events, when we ask why something happened, we see causes for events in the world. We look for reasons why somebody died, a reason why a natural disaster happened, reasons why a good thing happened. These reasons we would often assign to actions performed by a thinking entity, something or someone that wanted something to happen.

Now let's think back to a discussion of early development in which I told you about the capacities of infants starting from a very early age. Recall that I told you that three-month-olds divide the world into agents and objects where small children explicitly assign motives to inanimate objects. So, for instance, three-month-olds will make a distinction between a hand that comes in, which would be an agent coming in and grabbing for an object, as opposed to a stick coming in poking the object. So as early as the age of three months, small children, infants, will start categorizing the world into agents and objects. Later, small children explicitly do this and talk about it. They explicitly assign motives to inanimate objects. For instance, developmental psychologists have observed that small children think a ball rolls downhill because it wants to, or rolls along a surface. In everyday life we as adults don't hesitate to think of everyday objects as having personalities. We say cars or machines have personalities, we even name our cars. We do things like say that a tea kettle's whistling is cheery, or perhaps the storm sounds ominous.

It might seem natural then that early humans might have applied such reasoning to the events of the natural world. You can see this kind of reasoning in its most elemental form in animist religions which attribute a spirit to living and non-living objects. So starting with this metaphor of conscious agency to natural events, now let's add our intensely social nature, our theory of mind, our desire to bond and form social structures.

We have big neocortex, and we dedicate considerable mental resources to understanding other's motivations and other's points of view. This attribution of motives to oneself and to others is a capacity that requires and is very much overlapping with what's called theory of mind. Remember I told you about what it was that was necessary for theory of mind, what brain capacity seemed to be required. The assessment of social scenarios requires activity in many brain regions. One suggested region has been, not a region, but a type of neuron that has been found in various parts of the brain, mirror neurons, and these have been observed in monkeys. These are neurons that fire both when a monkey performs a task and also when the monkey sees another monkey do that same task. That observation, as I've talked about before, suggests that the monkey's brain understands that there's something in common between his and her own actions and the actions of another monkey.

I've also talked about social communication, social communication which requires structures such as the amygdala. The amygdala is a brain structure that's intimately involved in deriving the emotional significance of objects and faces. So the amygdala seems to be critical in giving the brain access to knowledge of the mental states of others. As I've said, these forms of social complexity seem to be related to the size of the cerebral cortex. It seems to be that social cognition requires a lot of horsepower. So, if you look at what I called before the brain arms race, this ability to cooperate and also to compete with our fellow beings, may be a capacity that set the stage for forming religious mental constructs. So as a consequence, our big sophisticated brains are capable of imagining a God, Yahweh, or Allah, that is the cause of everything and judges us, yet who cannot be seen.

Ethologists and anthropologists have been very interested in this theory of mind and have looked for theory of mind in other animals and have tried to quantify it by saying well, how many levels of intention can be imagined. Remember I talked about Osa, the dog who had a model in her mind that her owner Chris thought that she couldn't walk downstairs. That would be a relatively simple theory of mind inference. Chris thinks I can't walk downstairs, so Chris has a belief about me. If we think about religious belief, these levels of reasoning can become far more complex. So, for instance, a basic component of many religions is a two-step inference. God thinks, step 1, that I should worship him. The details of most religions involve more steps of inference. Let's take Christianity as an example. We have to keep straight what we want along with the desires of God, Jesus, and the Holy Spirit, there are the teachings of the church, and also of course what our fellow churchgoers think. This becomes a very complicated business.

This level of inference is something that seems to be the providence of human beings and not of other species. So, for instance, chimpanzees have some amount of theory of mind, but not this secondary multistep theory of mind. So, for instance, recall that a subordinate chimp will prefer to go after a piece of fruit that the dominant chimp can't see. That chimp will only go for the fruit that is not visible to the dominant chimp. Another example, if you appear unwilling to give a grape to a chimp, it'll lose interest. But if you show that you're willing, but unable to give the chimp the grape, maybe it'll wait longer. Chimps make these simpler inferences with a brain that is less than one-third the weight of ours. So it appears that there's something about having a large brain that allows us to make these complicated inferences.

I should say that there's some observational evidence that chimpanzees seem to have some kind of belief that resembles in some really suggestive way religious belief in us. It has been observed that during thunderstorms some chimps will sway around with their hair standing on end, so they will go like this during a storm looking at the clouds and at the storm. This is an act that some people have interpreted as resembling a dance. What is that? Are the chimps superstitious or are they just afraid?

Another component of religious belief is the transmission of those beliefs from generation to generation. The idea that those specific ideas, for instance, to take an example of the Holy Trinity, these are ideas need to be transmitted from generation to generation. What this requires is language-based transmission, the idea that accumulated ideas could be modified allowing a doctrine and a dogma to be communicated and preserved from generation to generation. So these stories, these ideas, these concepts have to be kept in order, preserved, and given from generation to generation.

Given what I've told you about other animals, I've told you about dogs, I've told you about chimpanzees, for now it seems to be the case that humans are alone in having the basic mental tools, namely a theory of mind and language, to generate organized religion. We may not have always been the ones with this exclusive gift. If you look back in the record of human evolution, before our species made the leap to religious belief some tens of thousands of years ago with our ritual burials and our cave art symbolism, it's possible that there might have been such events as well in Neanderthals. Neanderthals are of course another branch of the human lineage, and they have done so as long as 100,000 years ago. There's some evidence that Neanderthals also had an element of religious belief.

That's a brief summary of the necessary conditions of religious belief, and now what I want to do is talk a little bit about the languages aspect. This is an aspect that is not so well understood neuro-scientifically, but I think it's a very important capacity to think about in terms of what makes religious belief possible. Here's a general observation. Our capacity for language allows our search for causes and effects to take on a new dimension in the form of narrative. Recall that I've talked about storytelling, of long stories as something that seems to be a feature of the human brain. Recall that I've talked about the hippocampus as something that's important for spatial navigation, and also seems to be important for declarative memory, for forming memories of facts and events, and indeed long stories. I've talked about memory palaces, for example.

Human beings are story telling narrating animals, and as such, we have developed complex explantations for a wide variety of daily experiences and problems of existence. One consequence of language then is the formation of narratives. This has been looked at as a way of generating stories about the brain, about the world, and in particular the sociologist Christian Smith has written a book called *Moral Believing Animals*. He suggested that human belief systems are a general phenomenon in which we form narratives. We place the world into a coherent conceptual framework and we tell as story that gives meaning to daily experience. What Smith has specifically suggested is that these narratives have to have power. The power that he suggests that they have to have is the power of explanation. What has to happen in these narratives is they have to have a certain internal logic, they have to have internal consistency, and they have to meet some kind of criteria that tell us that those narratives are true.

Different kinds of narratives have different kinds of criteria for what makes them true. They have to feel true in different ways, and so I'd like to give you three examples of explanatory narratives, three very different examples, two of which are not religious at all. One kind of narrative Christian Smith calls "the capitalist prosperity narrative," and I will paraphrase his version of the capitalist prosperity narrative. It goes as follows. For most of human history the world's material production was mired in oppressive and inefficient economic systems such as primitive communalism, slavery, feudalism, mercantilism, and more recently, socialism and communism. In 18th-century Europe and America, however, enterprising men hit upon the keys to real prosperity: private property rights, limited government, the profit motive, capital investment, the free market, rational contracts, technological innovation. In short, economic freedom. And this capitalist revolution has produced more wealth, social mobility, and wellbeing, than any other system could possibly imagine or deliver.

We are familiar with this story. In the United States this is a commonly told story. It's a narrative that has a certain propulsive quality that guides a lot of political beliefs about what is so great about capitalism.

Here is another example of a narrative. This is a narrative that now accompanies the scientific enlightenment over the last centuries. This is a narrative than then is subscribed to in some form by many scientists and it goes as follows. For most of human history, people have lived in the darkness of ignorance and tradition, driven by fear, believing in superstitions. Ever so gradually, often at great cost, inventive men have endeavored better to understand the natural world around them. Centuries of such inquiry have eventually led to a marvelous scientific revolution that radically transformed our methods of understanding nature. We have come to possess the power to transform nature and ourselves. I should say that this scientific explanation relies on its own values. So we talked about the capitalist revolution and the capitalist prosperity narrative. The scientific narrative requires an observation of physical facts relying on physical observation to construct a model of the world that is tested against observations in nature. So again it's a narrative that has its own internal logic, its own checkpoints, if you will, for what makes it true or not. In the case of science, it's doing experiments.

The third example, and this comes back to our topic today, is finding meaning in the experience of living. The narrative that Smith proposes goes like this, this is the Christian narrative. A personal, loving, holy God created the heavens and Earth for His own glory, making humans in His very image, and establishing a relationship of care and friendship with humanity. Tragically, however, humans in pride have chosen to rebel against and reject God, the source of all life and happiness, thus plunging the world into all manner of evil, death, and spiritual blindness. But the love and grace of God is more powerful and determined than the sin of humanity, so through Israel, God continued His covenant and relationship to redeem the world from its sin.

That is a narrative that many people subscribe to that they hold quite dear. I've given you these three narratives. These narratives have very different rules, and very different goals. Any eventual neuro-scientific explanation of how we form narratives is likely to address them in similar ways, at least the part in which we think about how narratives lead us to form a belief and to hold a story close, to believe a story. I should also say that these narratives are not necessarily conflicting with one another because they have, as I mentioned, different internal standards of what's true or what sticks. For example, let's think of a scientific point of view of creation. How exactly would an omniscient omnipotent being run the world? One point of view is well, God would, in fact, put every detail in place. But another point of view might be that in fact the Lord works through amazing processes like natural selection and brains. So rather than having to stick fingers into everything from moment to moment, perhaps the way that creation works is by launching natural processes. The philosopher and poet Goethe said, "What kind of God would it be who only pushed the world from the outside?"

So if you put yourself in the point of view of what science can and can't do, it's not necessarily that neuroscience reduces spiritual life to something electrochemical. In this respect neuroscience is like other areas of science. Neuroscience is a way of understanding more deeply the world around us. In fact, it's possible for a scientist to also be deeply religious. For example, the current director of the United States National Institutes of Health is a man named Francis Collins. Dr. Collins is deeply religious, and also there are some neuroscientists whom I know who are also deeply religious and, in fact, committed Christians. One can imagine that for many of them, scientific research, the understanding in the world, is itself a form of worship.

Let's summarize what I've talked to you about in this lecture. I've said that meditative states, going back to the beginning, can trigger a variety of brain responses. I've pointed out these responses can include unusually high levels of whole brain synchrony and also enhanced attention related brain activity. In other words, spiritual experiences change your brain state. Religion itself requires other capacities, capacities that I've talked about in previous lectures, specifically theory of mind and a tendency and ability to identify conscious agents behind events and to then construct narratives about those events.

In the next lecture, the final lecture, what I would like to do is turn to a very general subject, the subject of happiness. I'd also like to take that as a launching point to describing how we might study the brain in the future and where neuroscience might go in explaining previously hard to explain phenomena.

Happiness and Other Research Opportunities
Lecture 36

It turns out that you never adapt to commuting to work. ... It's always going to make you, on average, a little bit less happy.

Surveys on happiness tell us some interesting things—for example, that happiness is strongly dependent, not on income, but on *relative* wealth. Happiness also is stable over time, despite the fact that our life circumstances obviously change. On whether major life events make us happy or unhappy in the long term, findings are somewhat surprising. Being married is correlated with happiness, but having children, according to these surveys, doesn't make us any happier.

Many results seem to be consistent with the concept of the hedonic treadmill: the idea that happiness seems to adapt and to have a set point. The general concept is that events that affect happiness are mostly temporary, so people quickly adapt back to hedonic neutrality. But some circumstances are reliably associated with unhappiness or with happiness. Affiliation with a religious or political group increases happiness, for example. But it turns out that you never adapt to commuting to work. It's always going to make you a little cranky.

Another principle is that one person may have many set points. At one stage of your emotional awareness, you might have different components of well-being, and these can move in different directions over life. These components not only vary over time but also in response to persistent positive or negative events and factors. Finally, our ability to adapt to events seems to vary by individuals. Strategies for increasing happiness in the face of this hedonic treadmill include the following:

- Finding ways to beat adaptation by experiencing frequent small events that are less likely to "adapt out" than one large event that then leads to a return to the set point.

- Focusing on positive events.

- Identifying character strengths and using them.

- Remembering to be grateful.

What's missing in this discussion is a good explanation of neuroscientific mechanisms, biological mechanisms, of what determines happiness. Accidental discoveries from neuroscience are relevant to this discussion of happiness. There are some surprising ways in which neuroscience could be useful. Current research is altering technologies that allow us to probe and study the brain in ways that we previously could not. Modern molecular biology methods allow us to alter the functions of neurons, build viruses that drive the expression of some proteins in neurons, and even cross synapses.

Technology similar to that used to locate seizure areas can be applied to develop brain-machine interfaces, like neural prosthetics. It's possible to achieve some crude degree of control over an artificial limb by decoding a person's motor commands. What that suggests is that technologically, it may become possible someday to restore some degree of function using brain-machine interfaces.

Other new fields are optogenetics, a means of manipulating a neuron by having it express its protein genetically and then applying light, and connectomics, the idea of deciphering and reconstructing an entire circuit: the connections, their physical arrangement, and the biochemical details.

All these technologies are at the cutting edge. It's reasonable to say that it's within reach for us to start understanding, at all levels, ranging from cognition and behavior to cells and circuits, what our brains are doing when we learn, when we love, and when we experience everyday life. ∎

Questions to Consider

1. What factors influence the hedonic treadmill? What major factors in your life seem likely to affect your happiness in the long run?

2. How do you imagine the new technologies described in this lecture (and yet undiscovered technologies) will affect the study of the brain?

Happiness and Other Research Opportunities
Lecture 36—Transcript

Welcome back. Throughout this course we followed our brains over many aspects of life, everyday aspects, unusual aspects. Now for this last lecture what I'd like to do is talk about a very every day aspect of brain function, one that's important to many of us, yet about which there's not that much hard neuroscience. That is namely, happiness. Because there's not that much I'll start by addressing the state of the neuroscience in this area of research, and then I'll move on to the kinds of problems that neuroscience could address in the future, not just this area, but also other areas as well.

If we think about problems we look to science to solve, we often think of diseases, in the case of neuroscience, aging, Parkinson's, autism and so on. But early in this course I claimed that neuroscience concerns much more. I claimed that it was relevant to everyday life. Today what I'd like to do is start by considering an everyday sort of problem, general happiness. Recall that I introduced lectures ago the topic of homeostasis and stress, and I talked about the fact that our brains often are trying to get us back to an even keel. That even keel in the case of emotional satisfaction changes over time and that is the measure of happiness. Obviously everyone would like to be happy. At least in the United States there's a major emphasis on happiness. It's even enshrined in the Declaration of Independence as an inalienable right, "life, liberty, and the pursuit of happiness."

So let's start by asking a question. How would you survey happiness? Well, the method perhaps is not surprising; you call people and ask them how happy they are. You ask them questions like, how satisfied are you with your life as a whole these days? Are you very satisfied, pretty satisfied, not very satisfied, or not at all satisfied? Questions like that. Then ask about a bunch of other stuff. Ask people about their income, their marital status, their hobbies. After asking all these questions, when people have this information, they take it from a significant sample and that typically requires thousands of people—then the researchers try to figure out what kinds of answers are more likely to come from happy people than from unhappy people. So the idea here is to identify life factors that change whether people report that they're happy.

Obviously one could come up with objections to this kind of research and I'll come back to that a little bit later, but this fundamentally is how one surveys happiness, how one measures it. When we look at these surveys the surveys tell some interesting things, some of which are kind of surprising. In the United States the results of happiness surveys show that happiness differences are not strongly dependent on income. So, above a certain level of income there seems to be not much difference in how happy people are. More money makes you more happy, which perhaps is not surprising, but what perhaps is surprising is that your minimal needs seem to be met, at least in regard to happiness, by about $30,000-per-year of income. It seems to be not that much compared with people who can often be very rich in societies as varied as the United States. But the determinant seems to be relative wealth; relative to one's neighbors, relative to what one had fairly recently. So that's one feature of happiness.

Another feature of happiness is that happiness has this curious property of being stable over time. There was one survey done following Germans over a 17-year-period following the same people over time. In the survey, only 24 percent of them changed significantly from the start of the survey to the end of the study over a long period of time. And only 9 percent of them changed a lot. So this again is a case where, getting back to the homeostatic idea, there seems to be relatively little change in happiness over long periods of time, despite the fact that our life circumstances can obviously change a lot over a period of say, 17 years.

So one principle that has come out of these data and other data is that there seems to be some comparison that we make that goes like this. It's not that we're comparing our lives with other possibilities, for instance like in a store, but more like it's comparing what you have to what you already own, or perhaps to what your friends have. So as I mentioned, there seems to be a factor of relative income that comes into these happiness surveys. Recall Barry Schwartz the psychologist who wrote a book called *The Paradox of Choice,* and what he pointed out is that people tend to be less satisfied with their decisions when they choose among many options compared with only a few options. So perhaps comparisons in general, perhaps tend to invite regret.

We can ask another question about happiness. Do major life events make us happy or unhappy in the long term? So, for example, we can ask whether life circumstances such as paralysis or blindness make us unhappy in the long term. There are some interesting phenomena here that are perhaps a little bit surprising. One finding is that blindness doesn't make people less happy. If you're blind you're no less happy on average than if you have your vision. Another example is lottery winners, and this is a very well known result. Something that's kind of counterintuitive, which is that you might imagine that if you win the lottery you'll be happier, and this is of course a common joke, oh if I won the lottery I'd be so much happier. It turns out that if you take lottery winners and surveyed their happiness at some time after their lottery win, they're not any happier than people who did not win the lottery. This experiment has even been done with proper controls where you compare people who play the lottery with equal frequency who play the lottery and win versus play the lottery and lose. There's not a difference in average happiness, and so it appears that something that is obviously as happiness inducing as winning the lottery, doesn't change average happiness.

There are other factors. Another factor is being married. So it turns out that being married is correlated with happiness. If you're married, you're more likely to be happy, you're happier on average than if you're not married. So that's one finding that comes out of these surveys. But having children, according to these surveys, doesn't make you any happier. People who are married with children and married without children are equally happy. So these kinds of results come from these surveys, and there are a lot of these different findings. It turns out that there are some general principles that seem to come out of these surveys. I've given you just a little laundry list of findings, and many of these surveys seem to be consistent with the concept that psychologists talk about called "the hedonic treadmill."

"Hedonic treadmill," that's sort of fancy sounding. What the hedonic treadmill refers to is the idea that our happiness seems to adapt and seems to have a set point, and the general concept goes as follows. Good and bad events that affect our happiness do so mostly temporarily. So, as a result, people are temporarily affected by an event, but they quickly adapt back to hedonic neutrality, wherever they were before the event happened. What this implies is that individual and societal efforts to increase happiness are, in fact, very difficult to make succeed. Some people have said well, maybe those efforts to increase happiness are doomed to failure. That's not quite right. So even though it's the case that some events will make us more happy or less happy, it turns out that there are some circumstances that I've listed that are reliably associated with unhappiness or with happiness. So, for instance, an example is chronic pain. It turns out that the vast majority of chronic pain sufferers are unhappy, and in fact, many are even depressed. Another example is commuting to work. It turns out that you never adapt to commuting to work. You can commute to work for as long as you like, but it's always going to make you, on average, a little bit less happy. So those are examples of events that alter your set point and then the set point still stays high or low.

So the hedonic treadmill hypothesis is one that requires modification. And if you look at some of these survey results and the ways that people turn out, you can find modifications, exceptions, and principles by which we have to start thinking a little bit differently about this central idea of the hedonic treadmill. One idea that has come out of subsequent surveys is that people have different set points. So individuals have different levels of intrinsic happiness and that those levels of happiness are partly dependent on their temperaments. I've talked about personality in this course. I've said that temperament is a partly inheritable trait. As it turns out, like temperament, happiness is also partially inheritable. Like personality, about 50 percent of the variation of the population of happiness is inheritable and that's based on, for instance, studies of identical twins and so on. Like personality there seems to be something similarly somewhat heritable from parents to children.

Another principle that comes out of the studies is that a single person may have multiple happiness set points. At one point in your life or at one stage of your emotional awareness you might have different components of wellbeing such as pleasant emotions, unpleasant emotions, and life satisfaction. These can move in different directions over life. So, for instance, at one point in your life you might have a very different level than another. In fact, another finding is that these wellbeing set points, this sense of happiness or wellbeing, can change over some conditions in a lasting fashion. So not only can it vary over time, it can vary in response to persistent positive events and factors, and these include, for instance, marriage. As I mentioned before, on average, married people are happier than unmarried people. Another factor that comes up is churchgoing people. So, people who go to church regularly are, on average, happier than people who don't go to church. This even pertains to, for instance, political affiliation. It turns out that Republicans are, on average, more happy than Democrats. This doesn't have very much to do with specific political beliefs, it turns out that it doesn't matter whether you're a liberal or a moderate, conservative or a moderate, there's something about your personal affiliation that makes you more happy. That could be correlated with other factors such as where you live, whether you live in an urban or a rural area, but yet, the correlation is there.

There are also persistent negative factors that affect our happiness negatively; one is the converse of finding a life partner and that is when you lose a spouse. So when your spouse dies, that reduces your happiness and that again is persistent. Likewise, and perhaps similarly, divorcing someone also is a source of a decrease in happiness that again does not adapt out. There are other examples of events that lead to decreases in happiness, one is unemployment. If you're unemployed your happiness decreases and then stays decreased. I've already mentioned disability and chronic pain, again, factors that decrease happiness, as well as commuting to work. One common thread that runs through these events is that all these events seem to be events that don't adapt and if you think about them, are events that seem like that would be hard to adapt to. So they are events of which we are reminded all the time. So that seems to be a feature that is shared by these kinds of events that can alter our set point up or down.

Finally there's a principle that comes out of research which is that our ability to adapt to events seems to vary by individuals. Some individuals adapt better than others, some individuals change their set point, others don't change their set point. They seem to be unaffected in their reactions to some external event. These are principles that modify the basic hedonic treadmill idea. In the face of this, can we think of strategies for increasing happiness in the face of this hedonic treadmill, in the face of this adaptive principle? One general principle that comes out of these surveys and seems to be the case for many of these factors is that one general principle is that in order to become happier on average, one can do so by finding ways to beat the adaptation. You can beat adaptation. So instead of having a large event and then it adapts out, another way you can beat adaptation is by having frequent small events. These frequent small events are less likely to adapt out than one large event that then leads to a return to the set point. So here are some examples.

The frequency of sex turns out to be, on average, something that makes a person more happy, frequently, and is, in fact, a more effective factor than socializing with friends. Another factor that seems to be good for happiness is sleep. Having a good night of sleep turns out to be a major determinant of happiness. It's, in fact, a better determinant of happiness than household income. So it's better to have a good night of sleep than to make more money. Another example is daily routine. You might have your opinions about daily routine, but in fact, it turns out that having a regular daily routine is a better predictor of happiness than having a variety of experiences. Another feature of life that seems to increase happiness is setting and achieving small realistic goals, in fact, on a daily basis.

Let's turn to another set of factors that seem to affect happiness. I'll start with a Charles Dickens quote, and the quote goes as follows, "Reflect on your present blessings of which every man has many, but not on your past misfortunes, of which all men have some." This quote can be exemplified by the following kinds of things. Surveys have shown, and interventional techniques have shown, that there are certain kinds of things that you can do to make your happiness greater on average. One is to focus on positive events. So for instance, to write down three good things that happen in a particular day, explain what caused each of them. This turns out to reduce symptoms of mild depression and the effects can last for months. Another is to identify character strengths and then to use them. That's something that seems to increase happiness. Finally, another thing that seems to increase happiness is to be remember to be grateful. I know that sounds a little bit treacly, but the advice is as follows. The intervention that seems to work is to write down five things for which you are thankful for. Writing down these five things leads to more positive feelings and fewer negative feelings. It's not quite putting up posters of kittens, but certainly it's a strategy that seems to work and has been demonstrated to work.

Now let's think briefly about the possible flaws in this work. These surveys are, of course, subject to objections. One objection is that the results of these surveys depend a little bit on how the question is asked. For instance, when people are asked to list activities that they particularly enjoyed overall, if they're just asked to list them, spending time with my kids comes up at the top of the list. But if you ask them then to describe how they felt during each of their activities in the previous days, interacting with children seems to be about as rewarding as doing housework or answering email. Which suggests the idea that children are somehow more rewarding in theory than in practice.

So let's summarize now what principles of happiness have come out of these psychological studies. One principle is that self-reported happiness has a set point that has a strong inborn component. Most life events, good or bad, tend to only have transient effects. The exception seems to be events of which one is reminded persistently, having a life partner, commuting to work on the negative side, chronic pain on the negative side. Conversely, a wide variety of events adapt out. So, for instance, increases in income and wealth, and having children, and when we make comparisons they tend to be to others around us who are right around us as opposed to comparisons over long periods of time. Perhaps because of adaptation, this hedonic treadmill can be beaten with many small events, but not big blockbuster events. In general, one interesting feature that comes out, for instance in the lottery example, is that we're bad at predicting what will make us happy in the long term. The lottery is one example, having children is another example. Although of course an objection could be made that maybe there are other things that are important besides being happy.

It turns out that a more accurate answer about what's going to make you happy can come from interrogating another person. So for instance if you're trying to determine whether you're going to be happy with a job decision or getting married or having children, a good strategy is to find someone who's like you and ask that person well, you made that decision, how happy did that make you? That turns out to be a way of getting a more accurate sense of these long-term effects on our happiness.

I did touch on one caveat in all of these studies which is the direction of causality. For instance, I mentioned that churchgoers are happier. Are they happier, or do they live under different demographic conditions? Maybe they live in places where, in fact, the environment is likely to make someone happier. Maybe they live in places where they don't commute as much. Does marriage make a person happier, or do happier persons get married? So another caveat is that happiness can be defined in different ways. So, for instance, asking about life satisfaction gives somewhat different responses. Are you happy about your children? Are you pleased, or do you regret the fact that you had children. And these can give different answers.

One thing you may have noticed in this discussion I've given of happiness, which I think does have practical implications, is that despite their practical implications, one thing that's missing is a good explanation at a mechanistic level. A lack of neuro-scientific mechanisms, biological mechanisms, of what it is that determines happiness. You might imagine that if we were trying to use neuroscience to understand everyday life, you could imagine that a way to increase happiness might be at the top of our list of problems to solve. But neuroscience is not currently at that place, and neuroscience doesn't always move in predictable directions. So right now, neuroscience research is not at that place. What's interesting is that there are accidental discoveries that have come from neuroscience that, in fact, are relevant to this discussion of happiness and so it's possible to start thinking about, well, how could neuroscience start leading us to understand happiness a little bit better? It turns out that there are some surprising ways in which neuroscience could be useful.

Let's think about one of these examples: deep brain stimulation. Recall that I talked about deep brain stimulation before in the context of treatments for Parkinson's disease. Deep brain stimulation in general began as a chance discovery by neurosurgeons who accidentally ruptured a blood vessel and inadvertently got rid of a patient's tremor. This eventually evolved into a more mild treatment not killing tissue, but stimulating it. In the end the treatment for Parkinson's disease was deep brain stimulation of the subthalamic nucleus. This is a pretty crude treatment, so even though this is state of the art, it's a pretty crude treatment because it stimulates, or perhaps even blocks, all of the cells in some region of the brain, in this case of the subthalamic nucleus. In fact, it's odd if you think about this. Stimulating a brain region would produce the same effect as a lesion. Stimulation, after all, doesn't kill brain tissue permanently. In fact, when the treatment is stopped, the effects disappear. So maybe stimulation has a jamming effect on the subthalamic nucleus. This could happen if stimulation interferes with impulses that are generated in or passed through the subthalamic nucleus. So, in fact, it's a fairly odd treatment.

Let's come to happiness. Recall that there are odd side effects that come from deep brain stimulation. All the near-miss regions, think about what I talked about before when talking about mood, these unexpected consequences in which, for instance, if you miss by a few millimeters you get deep depression or intense mania. Mucking around in the core of the brain leads to, for instance, mania in the case of euphoria, nonstop talking, grandiose delusions, increased sexual drive. All of these things that when people talk about these methods are so-called "neuropsychiatric side effects." If you look in the literature you can find apathy, hallucinations, compulsive gambling, cognitive dysfunction, as well as these changes in mood. All of these typically arise from incorrect placement or calibration of the stimulator.

But wait a minute, these side effects maybe are themselves very important. As I've mentioned before, the brain stem and midbrain are incredibly crowded places, jam-packed places. When it comes right down to it, we don't yet have a real idea of what a lot of these regions do. What that means is that neuroscience is in discovery mode in functions that seem to be as fundamental for our happiness as mood. There is, therefore, a major challenge and a major opportunity to start understanding these deep brain structures. Indeed, scientists have found all kinds of possibilities. They found that deep brain stimulation might even be useful for treating epilepsy or Tourette's syndrome.

Someday deep brain stimulation might be designed rationally based on what we know to be the functions of these various brain regions. But right now we seem to be limited by our basic knowledge of brain function. So when faced with the results of something like deep brain stimulation, we go and we poke things. What we've discovered is that when it comes to understanding how these core brain regions work, we seem to have a long way to go. Let me pose to you this question. How are we ever going to find out what these brain regions do? So far I've talked to you about lesion experiments, brain monitoring experiments, and therapies that seem state of the art, but we will probably someday look back at as being relatively primitive.

So what are we going to do? Well, let me now talk to you about research and about ways in which current research is altering how we think that we can probe the brain, technologies that allow us to probe the brain and study the brain in ways that we previously couldn't. So what I'd like to do is just take you on a very quick tour of current and future technologies, and how they might reveal principles of brain function more refined than what I've told you about before.

I've said that bits of brain are pretty crude. They have many cell types can you can find in just a cubic millimeter or even a few hundred cubic microns of tissue. Many of the methods are fairly crude. So one common motif that's in coming technologies for researchers is ways to refine our approaches to individual cells to start being able to ask questions, to manipulate function at a very fine level, even in intact brain tissue. Here's one example, genetics. I haven't talked very much in this course at all about the fact that it's possible in animals to alter gene expression. It is possible to take a mouse and to alter the function of a gene, or to add a gene, or to delete a gene. It's possible to change how and when genes are expressed. Modern molecular biology methods allow us to alter the function of neurons. It's even possible to build viruses that express protein that drive the expression of some protein in neurons, and even cross synapses. It's even possible to force expression through pathways in the brain and to get pathways in the brain labeled and to measure their function, to look at them, and to perhaps even manipulate them.

Another thing that we can do is something that is made possible by taking mice or other mammals, or flies, whatever your favorite model animal is, it's possible to change the molecular identity or function of a neuron. It's even possible to see the neuron. The way that this is possible is to make the neuron glow by adding a jellyfish protein. There's a jellyfish protein that goes by name of "green fluorescent protein," and from that name I think you can guess what it looks like. It is a green fluorescent protein that can be used to label a particular set of cells. It comes from jellyfish and we can use genetic methods to put it into animals and then to watch particular cells. You can, for instance, take cells and follow them over time. We can even engineer GFP, that's green fluorescent proteins' name, its abbreviation, and modify GFP and engineer it to start changing its brightness. So, for instance, if a neuron is active, when neurons fire action potentials, the ion calcium goes up inside the neuron and you can make a form of GFP that changes its brightness. It's possible then to engineer in a protein that alters its brightness and now we can even put it into neural tissue and now see the brightness of the cells get brighter or smaller and image brain function at the level of single neurons.

So in combination with other technologies, it's possible to image these proteins in the living animal. Recall earlier in this course I showed you a picture of a neuron that I imaged that I filled with fluorescent dye. It was a single Purkinje neuron, it was a type of neuron found in the cerebellum, a very complicated neuron. It's possible to use technologies like what I used to take that picture, a method called "two-photon microscopy," and it's possible to take that kind of technology, combine it with GFP, and start looking at these proteins to look at the structure of neural circuits, to look at circuits in+ a living animal.

For instance, let's look at this movie now. If we look at this movie, what we're looking at now is the brain of a living mouse. What this piece of brain tissue is doing is you can see this reconstruction rotating. These neurons are of the same type that I showed you in the other image where I filled the single neuron, now we're looking at hundreds of these neurons, hundreds of these Purkinje cells. The reason we can see them is that they are expressing this jellyfish protein, GFP. In particular in this particular movie it turns out that these neurons are expressing a form of GFP that changes its brightness in response to changes in calcium. So we can use, in fact, this modified protein to monitor activity in this neural circuit, and we can, in fact, monitor the whole circuit thinking. So just as I showed you before, as I've talked to you before about functional MRI, where you can monitor brain activity at the level of millimeter scale tissue, this is a method that promises in the future, and even in laboratories today, to allow us to monitor neural activity at the level of circuits, at the level of single neurons. So that's one example of what can be done with current technologies. This is a technology that's being developed and in use in laboratories around the world including my own laboratory.

It's one thing to monitor activity in a living animal. I just showed you a movie that comes from an intact mouse. It's even possible to combine this with other technologies that allow us to take these movies in an animal that is held still. So it's possible, for instance, to create environments that allow an animal to experience a virtual reality. So, for instance it's possible to even use simple consumer software like videogame software, to create a virtual environment that makes it possible to monitor neural like activity in a way that I just showed you in an animal navigating a virtual environment. For instance, it can be running a maze and you can have the animal run the maze and look at neural activity as the animal runs the maze. So that's another thing that's currently in use in laboratories today.

I've talked to you now about ways to monitor what neural tissue is doing, it's also possible to monitor what neural tissue is doing in a human patient and even stimulate neural tissue. Remember in past lectures I've talked about epilepsy patients. I've talked about how surgeons will put electrode arrays into epilepsy patients in order to monitor activity looking for seizure foci, places where seizures begin. It's possible to use similar technology to develop brain/machine interfaces, in particular things like neural prosthetics. So it's possible to take one of these beds of electrodes, so they often look like bed of nails, and you can take the bed of nails and then put it into the brain. You implant these beds of nails into brain tissue and even monitor activity through these electrode arrays and monitor what happens in the motor cortex of a person who has no control over their limbs, a paraplegic. It's possible to achieve some crude degree of control over an artificial limb in these people by decoding their motor commands to figure out what it is that they seem to have intended to do. What that suggests is the possibility that technologically it may become possible someday to, in fact, restore some degree of function, some degree of independence, to people using brain/machine interfaces.

In addition to monitoring activity, of course it's possible to activate tissue. I showed you some evidence in a past lecture about how one can drive current through the electrodes. Now let's combine some of the things that I've talked about here. I've talked about monitoring and manipulating neurons with electrodes. I've also talked to you about optical methods in which we can observe neural tissue and observe what the tissue is doing by putting in activity sensitive fluorescent proteins. One new field that's up and coming that has made its appearance on the neuroscience scene in the last few years is a field called "optogenetics." Now, optogenetics refers to a means of manipulating neurons by putting a protein in by having it express the protein genetically and then applying light. The way this can be done is by using a bacterial protein. This bacterial protein is called "channelrhodopsin," and it's a light harvesting protein that has nominally some functional similarity with the rhodopsin in the eye. Except in this case it's a light harvesting protein that's an ion channel. So you can get this protein expressed in neurons, you can use genetics to express it in specific neuron types, and get the ion channels to open when light comes in. There are even ion pumps that are light activated that can make a neuron less active. These proteins go by names such as "halorhodopsin" and "arch." These are proteins that can be driven to be expressed in only one cell type.

Let's come back to the example of deep brain stimulation for Parkinson's disease. I said that we don't really know exactly how it works, but there are recent results that show using these light sensitive proteins it's possible to now tickle particular neurons in the basal ganglia and say, well, does tickling that one do anything, does tickling that one do anything? It's emerging that a likely way that deep brain stimulation works is by specifically activating axons that come into the subthalamic nucleus. So it's possible to localize with some precision exactly which elements of a neural circuit are responsible for a behavior. So that's one thing that's starting to become possible with animal research.

Now that we've talked about specific cell types, this opens up another question. This other question is, well, how do we understand circuits? If we look at a block of brain tissue it's this impossible tangle. Remember I showed you images of neurons, and these neurons are embedded in this neural circuitry where everything is piled up on everything else. One field of study that has become very interesting is the field of connectomics. This is the idea of deciphering an entire circuit, reconstructing what all the connections are in a block of circuitry, the connections, their physical arrangement, and also the biochemical details of, say, what neurotransmitters are made by these neurons or perhaps what biochemical signaling machinery they have. This is a very big field that's up and coming and I think in the coming years we're going to be hearing a lot about connectomics as a field that's going to revolutionize neuroscience.

All these technologies are at the cutting edge. I've made a point of now introducing you to some ideas that go well beyond the methods that have been used over the last decades. Those methods are good methods, and most of what I've covered in this course is built upon previous knowledge gathered using those old methods. But let's just stop and think for a moment about what will be possible with these new methods. I think it's reasonable to say that it's within reach for us to start understanding, at all levels, ranging from cognition and behavior to cells and circuits, what our brains are doing when we learn, when we love, when we experience everyday life. To me this is a culmination of what people have been trying to do for decades, this field that seeks to understand the biology of who we are, the field of neuroscience.

Glossary

acetylcholine: A neurotransmitter whose functions include release from the ends of the final neurons in the parasympathetic nervous system.

action potential: A change in membrane potential arising at the axon hillock; it travels down the axon in an all-or-none fashion.

adrenal glands: Glands located above the kidneys; under stress, they release catecholamines and cortisol.

Alzheimer's disease: A degenerative neurological disorder characterized primarily by the loss of neurons in higher-order regions of the neocortex, limbic system structures, and specific reticular formation nuclei with widespread projections to the cortex.

amino acids: The building blocks of proteins; about 20 different kinds, akin to letters, exist. Unique sequences of amino acids are strung together to form a particular protein. That sequence determines the folded shape of that protein and, thus, its function.

amygdala: An almond-shaped nucleus beneath the rostral pole of the temporal lobe; involved in the processing of emotions, particularly fear.

androgens: A class of steroid hormones, including testosterone, with roles in aggression and sexual behavior in both sexes but most notably in males. (*See also* **anabolic hormones**.)

autonomic nervous system (ANS): A series of neural pathways originating in the hypothalamus, hindbrain, and brainstem and projecting throughout the body; it regulates all sorts of nonconscious, automatic physiological changes throughout the body. The ANS consists of the sympathetic and parasympathetic nervous systems.

axon: The process of a neuron specialized for the transmission of information; axons are the physical structures that connect different areas of the brain.

basal ganglia: A number of nuclei located subcortically in the forebrain. Many of the basal ganglia nuclei are involved in the extrapyramidal motor system.

biogenic amines: In the context of how the term is used in this course, it refers to the monoamine neurotransmitters dopamine, norepinephrine, and serotonin.

bipolar disorder (manic depression): An illness characterized by wide mood swings ranging from severe depression to expansive mania.

brain stem: A phylogenetically older area of the brain consisting of the midbrain, metencephalon, and myelencephalon.

central nervous system (CNS): The part of the nervous system comprising the brain and spinal cord.

cerebellum: Part of the metencephalon; involved in motor coordination and some cognitive functions.

cerebral cortex: The outer sheet or mantle of cells covering the hemispheres.

cochlea: Fluid-filled structure of the inner ear.

cognitive/cognition: Related to mental activities such as thinking, learning, and memory.

consciousness: The awareness of oneself and the world in a subjective sense.

dementia: A progressive mental deterioration.

dendrite: The part of the neuron that receives signals from other neurons. Dendrites tend to come in the form of highly branched cables coming from the cell body of a neuron.

depression: A disorder of "mood" characterized by an internal subjective state of hopelessness and despair.

dopamine: A neurotransmitter whose functions include a role in sequential thought (such that abnormal dopamine levels are associated with the disordered thought of schizophrenia), the anticipation of pleasure, and aspects of fine motor control.

emotion: A basic, physiological state characterized by identifiable autonomic or bodily changes.

epinephrine (a.k.a. adrenaline): Both a neurotransmitter throughout the brain and a hormone released in the adrenal gland during stress as a result of activation of the sympathetic nervous system.

estrogen: A class of female reproductive hormones.

evolution: When referring to biological systems specifically, a change in allele frequencies over time in a genetically continuous population of organisms.

frontal cortex: A recently evolved region of the brain that plays a central role in executive cognitive function, decision making, gratification postponement, and regulation of the limbic system.

gamma-aminobutyric acid (GABA): A major inhibitory neurotransmitter of the CNS, particularly of interneurons.

ganglion (pl. ganglia): A group of cell bodies in the peripheral nervous system; comparable to a nucleus in the central nervous system. Some structures in the central nervous system (e.g., basal ganglia) are also referred to as ganglia.

gene: A stretch of DNA that designates the construction of one protein.

glial cells: An accessory type of cell found in the nervous system. Glial cells support neuronal function by insulating the axons of neurons, indirectly supplying neurons with energy, scavenging dead neurons, and removing toxins from the extracellular space around neurons. (Contrast with **neurons**.)

glucocorticoids: A class of steroid hormones secreted during stress. They include cortisol (a.k.a. hydrocortisone) and synthetic versions, such as prednisone and dexamethasone.

glutamate: An excitatory neurotransmitter with critical roles in learning and memory. An excess of glutamate induces *excitotoxicity*, a route by which neurons are killed during various neurological insults.

gray matter: Areas where there are collections of neuronal cell bodies.

hippocampus: A brain region within the limbic system that plays a central role in learning and memory.

homeostasis: "Balance"; as used here, for example, balance between sympathetic and parasympathetic portions of the autonomic nervous system.

homunculus: Distorted figure of a "man" mapped onto brain regions in motor and somatosensory areas.

hormones: Blood-borne chemical messengers between cells.

hypothalamus: A limbic structure that receives heavy inputs from other parts of the limbic system; plays a central role in regulating both the autonomic nervous system and hormone release.

ion channel: Generally a protein that regulates the flow of ions, for example, across a membrane.

limbic system: A part of the brain most strikingly involved in emotion. Some major parts include the hippocampus, amygdala, hypothalamus, and septum.

magnetic resonance imaging (MRI)/functional magnetic resonance imaging (fMRI): A computer-assisted imaging that uses powerful magnets to create detailed images of soft tissue; functional MRI refers to the additional method of visualizing what areas of the brain are active or functional by their utilization of oxygen.

mutation: An error in the copying of a gene. Classically, mutations can take three forms: In *point mutations*, a letter in the DNA code is misread as a different letter. In *deletion mutations*, a letter is entirely lost. In *insertion mutations*, an extra letter is inserted.

natural selection: The process by which competition for limited resources causes the preservation or elimination of particular alleles.

neuron: Specialized cells of the nervous system.

neurotransmitter: Small molecules used by the brain to transmit signals across synapses from one neuron to another.

norepinephrine (a.k.a. noradrenaline): A neurotransmitter whose functions include release from the ends of the final neurons in the sympathetic nervous system, as well as a role in depression (with, most likely, a depletion occurring).

opioids: Naturally occurring "morphine-like" peptides in the brain.

orbitofrontal cortex: A part of the frontal lobe involved in impulse control, inculcation of cultural mores, and ability to appreciate the consequences of one's behavior.

oxytocin: The "love" molecule; a peptide hormone released by the hypothalamus; plays a role in a number of processes, including "bonding" in social animals.

parasympathetic nervous system: Part of the peripheral autonomic nervous system associated with "rest and digest" functions.

parietal lobe: A cortical lobe bordered by the central sulcus of Rolando anteriorly, the parieto-occipital sulcus posteriorly, and the Sylvian (lateral) fissure inferiorly.

Parkinson's disease: A neurodegenerative disease resulting from the loss of neurons in the substantia nigra of the midbrain; characterized by a resting tremor, abnormal posture, and paucity of normal movement.

perception: The mental process or act of awareness of an object or idea.

positron emission tomography (PET): An imaging method utilizing radioactive tagged glucose or oxygen to examine the metabolism and activity of neurons.

post-traumatic stress disorder (PTSD): A disorder characterized by anxiety and fear acquired because of a traumatic event.

prefrontal cortex: Part of the frontal lobe implicated in working memory.

protein: One of 5 categories of organic molecules present in all organisms. A protein consists of a chain of amino acids, the sequence of which is determined by information encoded in the genome. Proteins can act as enzymes and/or as structural components of organisms.

receptor: A protein that binds to other molecules, for example, a neurotransmitter; also the name given to various types of sensory neurons that respond to particular modalities, for example, rods and cones are visual sensory receptor neurons.

retina (neural retina): Multilayered sheet of neurons located at the back of the eyeball, and derived from the diencephalon in development.

retinal ganglion cells (RGCs): The neurons whose axons leave the eye to project to a variety of structures in the brain, including the lateral geniculate nucleus of the thalamus.

scientific method: The use of data collection, measurement, or other forms of experimentation followed by statistical analysis to determine objectively whether evidence exists to support or reject a scientific hypothesis.

sensation: The result of stimulation of sense organs; can also be a "feeling" in the somatosensory system.

serotonin: A neurotransmitter whose functions include a role in aggression, sleep onset, depression, and impulsivity.

stroke: Any acute neurological event related to impairment in blood flow or circulation in the central nervous system; can be hemorrhagic or ischemic.

sympathetic nervous system: The part of the peripheral autonomic nervous system involved with the "fight or flight" response.

synapse: Specialized contact between 2 neurons that allows one to send signals to the other.

synaptic plasticity: The dynamic property of synapses; believed to underlie learning and memory.

thalamus: A major structure of the diencephalon; composed of a number of individual nuclei, many of which project to the cortex, giving it the name "anteroom."

theory of mind: The understanding that other individuals have different thoughts and knowledge than you; most frequently used as a term in child development.

white matter: Axons; in the fresh brain, the myelin sheath surrounding axons gives it a "whitish" appearance.

Bibliography

The following two books provide a good introduction to neuroscience:

Aamodt, Sandra, and Sam Wang. *Welcome to Your Brain: Why You Lose Your Car Keys but Never Forget How to Drive and Other Puzzles of Everyday Life*. New York: Bloomsbury USA, 2009.

Bear, Mark F., Barry W. Connors, and Michael A. Paradiso. *Neuroscience: Exploring the Brain*. Baltimore: Lippincott Williams & Wilkins, 2006.

In addition, good resources exist for following current neuroscience news, including the magazine *Scientific American Mind* and several Web blogs:

Mind Hacks. http://www.mindhacks.com/.

The Neurocritic. http://neurocritic.blogspot.com/.

Neurophilosophy. http://scienceblogs.com/neurophilosophy/.

General Interest

Breedlove, S. M., Mark R. Rosenzweig, and Neil V. Watson. *Biological Psychology: An Introduction to Behavioral, Cognitive, and Clinical Neuroscience*. Ann Arbor, MI: Sinauer Associates, 2007. A college-level textbook on psychological phenomena treated from a neuroscientific point of view.

Gross, Charles G. *A Hole in the Head: More Tales in the History of Neuroscience*. Cambridge, MA: MIT Press, 2009. General essays on topics in the history of neuroscience, including trepanation, left-right asymmetry, and adult neurogenesis.

Linden, David J. *The Accidental Mind: How Brain Evolution Has Given Us Love, Memory, Dreams, and God*. Cambridge, MA: Belknap Press of Harvard University Press, 2008. A neuroscientist considers the brain not as a carefully engineered machine but, with all its imperfections and foibles, as the complex outcome of contingent events over the course of evolution.

Ramachandran, V. S., and Sandra Blakeslee. *Phantoms in the Brain: Probing the Mysteries of the Human Mind.* New York: Harper Perennial, 1999. A neurologist and a neuroscience writer together consider the strange quirks that emerge when the pain of a missing limb is caused by the lingering presence of its representation in the brain. [Suggested reading for Lectures 7, 8, and 9.]

Specific Topics

Aamodt, Sandra, and Sam Wang. "Tighten Your Belt, Strengthen Your Mind." *New York Times*, April 2, 2008, p. A27 (op-ed). [Suggested reading for Lecture 15.]

Basso, Olga. "Right or Wrong? On the Difficult Relationship between Epidemiologists and Handedness." *Epidemiology* 18 (March 2007):191–193. [Suggested reading for Lecture 21.]

Bauby, Jean-Dominique. *The Diving Bell and the Butterfly: A Memoir of Life in Death.* New York: Vintage, 1998. A memoir of locked-in syndrome; the basis for the film of the same title.

Blanke, Olaf, Christine Mohr, Christoph M. Michel, Alvaro Pascual-Leone, Peter Brugger, Margitta Seeck, Theodor Landis, and Gregor Thut. "Linking Out-of-Body Experience and Self Processing to Mental Own-Body Imagery at the Temporoparietal Junction." *Journal of Neuroscience* 25 (2005):550–557. [Suggested reading for Lecture 34.]

Buckner, Randy L. "Memory and Executive Function in Aging and AD: Multiple Factors That Cause Decline and Reserve Factors That Compensate." *Neuron* 44 (2004):195–208. [Suggested reading for Lectures 22 and 23.]

Chawla, Lakhmir S., Seth Akst, Christopher Junker, Barbara Jacobs, and Michael G. Seneff. "Surges of Electroencephalogram Activity at the Time of Death: A Case Series." *Journal of Palliative Medicine* 12 (2009): 1095–1100. [Suggested reading for Lecture 34.]

Colcombe, Stanley and Arthur F. Kramer. "Fitness Effects on the Cognitive Function of Older Adults: A Meta-Analytic Study." *Psychological Science* 14 (2003):125–130. [Suggested reading for Lecture 23.]

Damasio, Antonio. *Descartes' Error: Emotion, Reason, and the Human Brain.* New York: Penguin, 2005. [Suggested reading for Lectures 26, 27, and 28.]

Dehaene, Stanislas. *The Number Sense: How the Mind Creates Mathematics.* New York: Oxford University Press, USA, 1999. [Suggested reading for Lecture 32.]

Diamond, Adele, W. Steven Barnett, Jessica Thomas, and Sarah Munro. "Preschool Program Improves Cognitive Control." *Science* 318 (2007):1387–1388. [Suggested reading for Lecture 18.]

Doidge, Norman. *The Brain That Changes Itself: Stories of Personal Triumph from the Frontiers of Brain Science.* New York: Penguin, 2007. [Suggested reading for Lectures 7, 8, 12, and 13.]

Flynn, James R. *What Is Intelligence? Beyond the Flynn Effect.* New York: Cambridge University Press, 2009. [Suggested reading for Lecture 25.]

Gilbert, Daniel. *Stumbling on Happiness.* New York: Vintage, 2007. [Suggested reading for Lectures 10 and 36.]

Gopnik, Alison. *The Philosophical Baby: What Children's Minds Tell Us about Truth, Love, and the Meaning of Life.* New York: Farrar, Straus and Giroux, 2009. [Suggested reading for Lectures 18 and 19.]

Gradinaru, Viviana, Murtaza Mogri, Kimberly R. Thompson, Jaimie M. Henderson, and Karl Deisseroth. "Optical Deconstruction of Parkinsonian

Neural Circuitry." *Science* 324 (2009): 354–359. [Suggested reading for Lecture 36.]

Harris, Judith Rich. *The Nurture Assumption: Why Children Turn Out the Way They Do*. New York: Free Press, 2009. [Suggested reading for Lectures 18, 19, 20, 24, and 25.]

Kandel, Eric R. *In Search of Memory: The Emergence of a New Science of Mind*. New York: W.W. Norton & Co., 2007.

Katz, Bernard. *Nerve, Muscle and Synapse*. New York: McGraw-Hill, 1966. [Suggested reading for Lecture 4.]

LeDoux, Joseph. *The Emotional Brain: The Mysterious Underpinnings of Emotional Life*. New York: Simon & Schuster, 1998. [Suggested reading for Lectures 26, 27, and 28.]

Levitin, Daniel J. *This Is Your Brain on Music: The Science of a Human Obsession*. New York: Plume/Penguin, 2007. [Suggested reading for Lecture 32.]

Marcus, Gary. *Kluge: The Haphazard Evolution of the Human Mind*. New York: Mariner Books, 2009. [Suggested reading for Lectures 3 and 10.]

Panda, Satchidananda, John B. Hogenesch, and Steve A. Kay. "Circadian Rhythms from Flies to Human." *Nature* 417 (2002):329–335.

Risley, Todd R., and Betty Hart. *Meaningful Differences in the Everyday Experience of Young American Children*. Baltimore, MD: Paul H. Brookes Publishing Co., 1995. [Suggested reading for Lectures 18 and 19.]

Sacks, Oliver. *Awakenings*. New York: Vintage, 1999. [Suggested reading for Lectures 5 and 6.]

Sapolsky, Robert M. *Why Zebras Don't Get Ulcers*. New York: Holt Paperbacks, 2004. [Suggested reading for Lecture 16.]

Schacter, Daniel L. *Searching for Memory: The Brain, the Mind, and the Past*. New York: Basic Books, 1997. [Suggested reading for Lectures 12, 13, and 14.]

Schwartz, Barry. *The Paradox of Choice: Why More Is Less*. New York: Harper Perennial, 2005. [Suggested reading for Lectures 10 and 36.]

Smith, Christian. *Moral, Believing Animals: Human Personhood and Culture*. New York: Oxford University Press USA, 2009. [Suggested reading for Lecture 35.]

Snyder, Solomon H. *Drugs and the Brain*. Scientific American Library Series, vol. 18. New York: W.H. Freeman & Company, 1996. [Suggested reading for Lectures 5 and 6.]

Thagard, Paul. *The Brain and the Meaning of Life*. Princeton: Princeton University Press, 2010. [Suggested reading for Lectures 33 and 35.]

Notes

Notes

Notes

Notes